The New Politics of Medicine

The New Politics of Medicine

Brian Salter

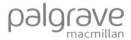

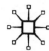
First published 2004 by
PALGRAVE MACMILLAN
Houndmills, Basingstoke, Hampshire RG21 6XS and
175 Fifth Avenue, New York, N.Y. 10010
Companies and representatives throughout the world

PALGRAVE MACMILLAN is the global academic imprint of the Palgrave
Macmillan division of St. Martin's Press, LLC and of Palgrave Macmillan Ltd.
Macmillan® is a registered trademark in the United States, United Kingdom
and other countries. Palgrave is a registered trademark in the European
Union and other countries.

ISBN 0–333–80112–1 paperback

This book is printed on paper suitable for recycling and made from fully
managed and sustained forest sources.

A catalogue record for this book is available from the British Library.

10   9   8   7   6   5   4   3   2   1
13 12 11 10 09 08 07 06 05 04

Printed and bound in China

This book is dedicated to my mother, father and John

Contents

List of figures and tables

Figures

Tables

List of abbreviations

AGMETS	Advisory Group on Medical Education and Staffing
AMA	American Medical Association
AMRC	Academy of Medical Royal Colleges
ASGB	General Syndicate of Belgium Physicians
BCAG	Bristol Heart Children's Action Group
BMA	British Medical Association
BVAS	Belgium Association of Medical Syndicates
BUPA	British United Provident Association
CAM	Complementary and Alternative Medicine
CCSC	Central Consultants and Specialists Committee
CCST	Certificate of Completion of Specialist Training
CHAI	Commission for Healthcare Audit and Inspection
CHC	Community Health Council
CHG	Community Hospitals Group
CHI	Commission for Health Improvement
CME	Continuing Medical Education
CMO	Chief Medical Officer of the Department of Health
CNAMTS	Caisse National de l' Assurance Maladie des Travailleurs Salaries
COPE	Committee on Publication Ethics
COPMeD	Conference of Postgraduate Medical Deans of the United Kingdom
CPPIH	Commission for Patient and Public Involvement in Health
COREC	Central Office for Research Ethics Committees
DHA	District Health Authority
DoH	Department of Health
DHSS	Department of Health and Social Security
DRG	Diagnostic Related Group
DTC	Diagnostic Treatment Centre
DTC	Direct to consumer advertising
FHSA	Family Health Service Authority
FDA	Federal Drugs Agency
GDC	General Dental Council
GKV	Gesetzliche Krankenversicherung
GMC	General Medical Council

GMS	General Medical Services
GPC	General Practitioners Committee of the BMA
GPR	General Practitioner Registrar
HA	Health Authority
HCSA	Hospital Consultants and Specialists Association
HCFA	Health Care Finance Administration
IHA	Independent Healthcare Association
IMSS	Instituto Mexicano del Seguro Social
JCC	Joint Consultants' Committee
JCHMT	Joint Committee on Higher Medical Training
JCHST	Joint Committee on Higher Surgical Training
JCPTGP	Joint Committee on Postgraduate Training for General Practitioners
JPAC	Joint Planning Advisory Committee
KNMG	Royal Dutch Society for the Promotion of Medicine
KV	Kassenärztliche Vereinigung
LHV	National Association of GPs (Netherlands)
LSV	National Association of Specialists (Netherlands)
LREC	Local Research Ethics Committee
MAC	Medical Advisory Committee
MMC	Monopolies and Mergers Commission
MMSAC	Medical Manpower Standing Advisory Committee
MCA	Medicines Control Agency
MEPP	Maintenance and Enhancement of Professional Performance
MMC	Monopolies and Mergers Commission
MRC	Medical Research Council
MREC	Multi-centre Research Ethics Committee
NCAOR	National Committee Relating to Organ Retention
NCSC	National Care Standards Commission
NCAA	National Clinical Assessment Authority
NDPB	Non-Departmental Public Body
NHSE	National Health Service Executive
NICE	National Institute for Clinical Excellence
NPM	New Public Management
NPSA	National Patients Safety Agency
NSF	National Service Framework
NTN	National Training Number
NWDB	National Workforce Development Board
PACT	Prescribing Analysis and Costs

PALS	Patient Advocacy and Liaison Service
PCG	Primary Care Group
PCI	Communist Party (Italy)
PCT	Primary Care Trust
PFI	Private Finance Initiative
PGMDE	Postgraduate Medical and Dental Education
PITY II	Patients Interring Their Young Twice
PMI	Private Medical Insurance
PMS	Personal Medical Services
PPP	Private Patients Plan
PPU	Private Patient Unit
PRHO	Pre-Registration House Officer
RBRVS	Resource Based Relative Value Scales
RCGP	Royal College of General Practitioners
RCOG	Royal College of Obstetricians and Gynaecologists
REC	Research Ethics Committee
RHA	Regional Health Authority
SAC	Specialist Advisory Committee
SHA	Strategic Health Authority
SHO	Senior House Officer
SpR	Specialist Registrar
SIFT	Special Increment for Teaching
SSN	Servizio Sanitorio Nazionale
STA	Specialist Training Authority
STC	Specialist Training Committee
SWAG	Specialist Workforce Advisory Group
VBS	Federation of Belgium Associations of Medical Specialists
WDC	Workforce Development Confederation
WNAB	Workforce Numbers Advisory Board

Introduction

In May 1998, the General Medical Council (GMC) ruled that two surgeons from Bristol Royal Infirmary were guilty of continuing to operate on children with heart defects when they knew their death rates were unacceptably high. In addition, a doctor manager was found guilty of failing to stop the operations after he had been alerted to the high mortality. Accompanied by intense media interest, these decisions launched an unprecedented period of politicisation for the medical profession, one where new power relationships were forged and others abandoned. Public trust in doctors appeared to be in the balance. Medical politics was unaccustomed both to such uncertainty and to such visibility. Traditionally, issues of power were handled informally and change was negotiated according to a timescale where decades were an appropriate unit of measurement. Suddenly this leisurely style was rendered obsolete by the mobilisation of public opinion against the profession and a rapid series of moves by the state to gain political advantage.

This book is about the context and consequences of that politicisation and above all about the continuities that mark out medical power as a distinctive political phenomenon. For the politics of medicine are driven by an enduring relationship between the profession, civil society and the state around which lesser political forces are obliged to coalesce. That relationship is reflected in cultural assumptions, hierarchies of social status, legal arrangements and institutions such as those of the National Health Service (NHS) which form part of the basic fabric of British political life. To suppose that the mere act of policy making can rearrange such a diverse constellation of forms of power, interlocked by habit and routine, is to misunderstand how the politics of medicine work. Like other forms of politics, they cannot be divorced from their context. Unlike most other forms of politics, that context endows the profession with unrivalled political resources.

The analysis of medical power therefore requires a theoretical approach which includes a systemic view of medicine's contribution to health politics, a mesa-level analysis of the engagement between policies, institutions and values, and a micro-level awareness of the political significance of the doctor–patient relationship. In pursuit of this ambitious (and difficult) synthesis the book draws on medical sociology, the sociology of knowledge and the public policy frameworks of political science in constructing its understanding of how the politics of medicine work. Medical power is theorised as a multifaceted phenomenon capable of operating simultaneously at numerous social and political levels. Therein lie its complexity, its strength and its fascination.

Given the nature of the guiding theory, the book has necessarily taken its data from diverse sources including conventional research findings, statistics wherever they are available, journal and newspaper reports and, most commonly, the policies, procedures and consultation documents of government, medical institutions and other participating agencies. The ready availability via the internet of policy documentation of all kinds has revolutionised the speed with which this material can be accessed, provided you know how to access them. In this respect, this book is indebted to my secretary Jenni Shand who regularly penetrated the most unpromising websites to obtain obscure but important material. Analysing the latter is a form of contemporary archive work in its own right. As has already been indicated, policy statements and their supporting guidance have to be placed within the appropriate context of power relations for their political significance to be properly understood. Examined in isolation or in their own terms policy materials have no analytical value. Once the context is established the details of the text can be explored to identify the way in which values, power relationships and forms of legitimation are expressed in policy terms. Thus, policy is viewed as a vehicle for enhancing our understanding of the underlying power struggle rather than as a literal reflection of political reality.

The details of that power struggle have also been accessed through a dialogue with key political actors. Senior members of the medical profession have generously given of their time to comment on the drafts of chapters, correct factual inaccuracies and tender their own views on the interplay of political forces. In return, the author has given generously of his time to provide the profession with advice by presenting papers at medical conferences and publishing in medical trade journals. Two outstanding figures of medical politics have been particularly helpful: Sir Donald Irvine and Sir Alexander Macara. More informally, but no less significantly, the book owes a debt to Professor Meg Stacey. Her seminal work on the GMC supplied an original intellectual inspiration and her personal introduction to senior medical figures an avenue for developing the reciprocal relationship just described.

The dominating theme of the book is the enduring nature of medical power. Chapter 1 provides the theoretical basis for this argument in terms of the contribution of medicine to the macrolevel relationship between medicine, civil society and state and the geology of the consequent political dynamic in British politics. Within this general context, the politics of medicine are played out in many arenas. Chapter 2 deals first with the evidence on the nature of the changing engagement between doctor and patient, the apparent reformulation of the relationship and then explores the extent to which change in this arena is characterised by underlying continuities. This theme is reiterated in Chapter 3 where the claims of patient empowerment are subject to the slide rule of political analysis and the test of access to the health policy community. As the instruments of the state, managers are an important part of the political equation of medicine and, as Chapter 4 argues, the extent to which they have gained and lost power is a measure of medical influence. Chapter 5 then deals with the heartland of medicine's political identity; the complex and largely inaccessible world of self-regulation where doctors hold sway over doctors. This provides the backdrop to the account in Chapter 6 of the state's assault on the medical stronghold and its ill-starred attempt to re-engineer its macro-relationship with the profession. The NHS is, of course, but part of medicine's tangled political story. Chapter 7 analyses how the ability of doctors to travel across the boundaries of the private and public health care sectors with relative impunity is assuming increasing political significance as those boundaries become ever more permeable. Finally, in the light of the traumatic events of the past few years, the apparent rise of the empowered patient and the production of numerous state policies for the regulation of doctors but few for the protection of battered managers, Chapter 8 reviews the balance of power between doctors on the one hand and patients, managers and politicians on the other. What, if anything, has changed in the politics of medicine?

1 Medicine, civil society and the state

Introduction

The politics of medicine are driven by a triangle of intersecting forces between the profession, civil society and the state. As the pressures at work within the triangle have changed and evolved, so also have the politics of medicine: adjusting, reformulating and seeking advantage. It is by no means a random political process but one guided by a fundamental problem of citizenship arising from civil society's legitimate expectations of the welfare state in general and the Health Service in particular. In responding to those expectations and to the political demands they represent, the state is dependent on the profession of medicine for the fulfilment of its responsibilities and promises to the electorate. Regardless of the rhetoric of politicians, doctors remain a necessary vehicle for the delivery of citizens' health care rights. Medicine, therefore, has both a political function and a bargaining position of systemic significance.

Drawing on international comparisons, the task of this chapter is to translate this general statement into a framework for the analysis of medical power. It begins with the problem of welfare citizenship as a key issue in a democratic polity such as the UK. What is the relationship between citizenship rights, the demand for health care, the role of the state and the position of medicine? Second, how can we best analyse the engagement between the control of medical knowledge, public trust and the regulatory institutions of the profession? Third, to what extent is the interdependence of medicine and the state manifest in terms of an enduring and resilient concordat? Finally, how responsive is that concordat to pressures for change and what forms does international experience suggest its reformulation can take?

1

Medicine and citizenship

Citizenship can be defined as a reciprocal relationship between the individual and the state. As citizens, individuals have rights which the state guarantees to fulfil and duties which they must carry out for the state. In his seminal work *Citizenship and social class* Marshall makes a distinction between the civil rights necessary for individual freedom, the political rights necessary for participation in the exercise of political power and social rights. For Marshall, social rights are 'the whole range from the right to a modicum of economic welfare and security to the right to share to the full in the social heritage and to live the life of a civilised being according to the standards prevailing in society' (Marshall, 1950: 5). Whereas civil and political rights are generally formulated in a negative way in terms of freedom from something, social rights require an active and interventionist state to give the formal status of citizenship a material foundation. Many discussions of social rights agree, with Marshall, that the means used by the state to meet its obligations to its citizens should be the welfare state. Access to state welfare services then becomes part of the practical status of citizenship, an integral part of citizenship expectations and an immutable political demand upon the state.

Within welfare state citizenship, health care rights play a central role. The 1946 Act establishing the National Health Service (NHS) stated that 'It shall be the duty of the Minister of Health ... to promote the establishment in England and Wales of a comprehensive health service ... The services provided shall be free of charge, except where any provision of this Act expressly provides for the making and recovery of charges' (Watkin, 1975: 140–1). The right to comprehensive free health care from the cradle to the grave had been born, and with it a new and powerful political dynamic. Significantly, neither the 1946 legislation nor its successor Act of 1977 actually defines the nature of health, illness or care: what is, and what is not, the responsibility of the state. Given that in creative hands the range of human conditions and requirements encompassed by these terms can be expanded almost indefinitely, the potential statutory scope of the Health Service is correspondingly unlimited. There is no necessary conflict between the statutory duties of the NHS and that most inclusive of definitions of health by the World Health Organisation in its Alma Ata declaration which asserts that health consists of a 'state of complete physical, mental and social well-being, not merely the absence of disease and infirmity'. Thus the UK has no 'core' definition of the citizen's social right to health care. The right to health is a negotiable political concept.

If health care rights are infinitely expandable, so also is the political demand that citizens can legitimately place on the state which has so generously bestowed these rights. It seems unlikely that British politicians were aware of the steamroller dynamic inherent in the foundation of the NHS and the political logic it was to impose on their successors. The calculation at the time was that there existed a finite amount of ill-health in the land, that this could be reduced by improved health care and that thereafter the maintenance of the good health of the population would be a relatively simple matter. Disillusionment was swift. In 1948–49, the year following the creation of the NHS, the number of prescriptions tripled and a huge demand for the now free medicines, dentures and spectacles became manifest. The mistake had been to see health care demand as a function of an identifiable concept of 'population health' rather than as a function of citizenship.

Several factors have acted to expand the significance of this citizenship problem for the state. As an established ideology, welfare state values act to prevent any questioning of the right to health care (however defined) and hence any serious examination of the political issues generated by it. It is assumed instead that the social rights of citizenship can be increased but not diminished: as Enoch Powell once put it, that 'no social benefit once conferred can ever be withdrawn'. Once a new health care right has been added to the existing list required by 'the healthy citizen' it immediately becomes part of the welfare orthodoxy and a useful benchmark for potential additions to that list. No putative social right can *a priori* be regarded as off-limits nor can the social rights domain of British citizenship ever be regarded as complete. The effect of this ideological 'ratchet' on the political culture in health care is twofold. For citizens, it means they are encouraged to register their demands in the present areas of provision, to expect new health care rights to emerge and to accept them as legitimate when they do. For the state, it means that any attempt it may make to reduce health care demand through a reformulation of citizenship which results in fewer rights will face entrenched ideological opposition.

That opposition is embedded in a powerful political constituency of welfare professionals, client lobby groups and academics, ready for rapid mobilisation on any given health issue (Klein, 1993).

During the long winter of Conservative rule, it was the fear of left-wing commentators that, as one put it, there would be difficulty 'in upholding the civilising influence of the welfare state against a determined Conservative drive to define the limits of welfare' (McCarthy, 1989: 8). Although the Conservatives proved to be less competent barbarians than the left had feared, and although the growth of expenditure on the welfare state continued to rise (if more slowly), what Thatcherism did achieve was the ideological incorporation of consumerism into British welfare citizenship.

At the heart of the New Right values of the Thatcher era is the concept of citizens as consumers activating their right to welfare through the exercise of choice in the market place. In order for that choice to be efficient and effective, appropriate information must be provided to the consumer, and the power of welfare professionals to interfere with the operation of the market suitably curtailed. Public bureaucracies must shrug off their monolithic and paternalistic image and evolve into transparent, responsive, 'enabling authorities'. Overall, in the new scheme of things 'citizenship relates less to participation in the public realm than to consumption in the private realm' (Walsh, 1995: xviii). Nowhere in any of this is there the suggestion that citizen rights are being reduced. Certainly, the way in which the rights are to be expressed is redefined, but the state retains its responsibilities for ensuring the delivery of welfare to its citizens. As Saunders points out, the 'privatised mode does not entail a withdrawal of the state but only a change in the form (and perhaps to some extent the scale) of its intervention in everyday life' (Saunders, 1993: 65). The assumption is that the bulk of the finance will remain public, that much of the provision will be private and that regulation will become more sophisticated. Gamble may be right that a central goal of Thatcherism was 'to discredit the social democratic concept of universal citizenship rights guaranteed and enforced through public agencies, and to replace it with a concept of citizenship rights achieved through property ownership and participation in markets' (Gamble, 1988: 16). If so then clearly it failed since in the case of welfare those markets remain heavily state subsidised and regulated.

What Thatcherism did achieve is welfare citizenship with a distinctive consumer edge. Rather than reducing rights, it actually increased them by inventing new ways in which citizens could demand that their legitimate expectations be met within the framework of state responsibilities. The consumption of health care remained a collectively organised form of state provision but citizens were encouraged to behave as consumers with market power and product choice. Thus in the early 1990s, for example, rights-based Patients Charters were promulgated: creating, monitoring and politicising new and highly visible areas of patient demand (Department of Health, 1992, 1995). Citizens could now expect not just more health care, but better quality health care also.

The expansion of health care rights has never been matched by an equivalent increase in the supply of health care resources generated by the citizenship duty of the payment of the taxes from which the Health Service is funded. As a consequence, the demand–supply mismatch has always been a fundamental feature of the NHS. (Perhaps because of this, its critical political significance for the continuing power of medicine is frequently underestimated. Familiarity has, as it were, bred analytical neglect.) In the long and contorted history of the NHS, its political manifestation has taken various forms and includes: rationing, priority setting, cost-containment, under funding and, most commonly, waiting lists. All of these issues constitute different ways of describing and presenting the consequences of the citizenship problem. Their variety is a measure of the numerous facets of the problem, their permanence a tribute to the state's need for a means to manage it.

Given the hegemony of the welfare state ideology, the state has never been able to manage the demand–supply mismatch explicitly since public rationing is a denial of someone's, or some group's, health care rights. By definition, such mechanisms can be immediately challenged so that, as Mechanic observes 'explicit rationing is inevitably unstable because of the ability of small groups to evoke public sympathy and support in contesting government decision making ... [thus] pushing the health system toward more flexible implicit approaches' (Mechanic, 1995: 1658). In this situation, covert rationing by doctors of the health care demand from civil society becomes the only available option. But if the medical profession is to provide the state with an avenue of escape from the citizenship cul-de-sac of its own making, clearly a political exchange is required. Klein has elegantly described the consequent basis of what he calls 'the politics of the double bed' that underlay the foundation of the NHS,

> it created a situation of mutual dependency. On the one hand the state became a monopoly employer: effectively members of the medical profession became dependent on it not only for their own incomes but also for the resources at their command. On the other hand the state became dependent on the medical profession to run the NHS and to cope with the problems of rationing scarce resources in patient care. (Klein, 1990: 700)

A high level and mutually beneficial concordat was thus established.

However, for the arrangement to work, a further contract was necessary between medicine and civil society to ensure that the public trusted and accepted the clinical (and rationing) decisions of doctors. This centred on the principle of self-regulation which, in the words of the Merrison Report, is 'a contract between the public and the profession, by which the public go to the profession for medical treatment because the profession has made sure it will provide satisfactory treatment' (Merrison Committee, 1975: 3). If the profession does not or cannot fulfil its part of the bargain, then the state is obliged to reform medical regulation in order to restore public confidence. As Merrison emphasises, 'The legislature – that is, Parliament – acts in this context for the public, and it is for Parliament to decide the nature of the contract [between medicine and the public] and the way it is executed' (Merrison Committee, 1975: 5). If the state fails to act and as a result does not meet the terms of its contract with its citizens (the delivery of health care rights), it must expect to lose their support. It is thus in the very nature of this ménage á trois that difficulties with one relationship inevitably impact on the other two.

In summary, then, the three contracts between medicine, civil society and the state interlock to form a triangle of forces based on a mutual exchange of political benefits (Figure 1.1).

The political benefits are as follows:

- as members of a modern welfare state, citizens receive their health care rights from the state delivered to an appropriate standard by medicine;

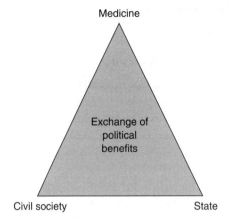

Figure 1.1   The triangle of political forces

- the welfare duty of the state is thus fulfilled, it gains the respect of its citizens whilst relying on the medical profession to manage the inevitable tensions between the demand for health care and the available supply;
- by fulfilling its obligations to both, the profession receives the trust of the citizenry, the privilege of self-regulation from the state, and a consequent set of social and economic advantages.

Medicine therefore derives its political strength from its historic ability to facilitate the solution to a central citizenship problem. But, in theoretical terms, how can we translate this understanding of medicine's macro-level advantage into a mesa-level analysis of its institutional power?

Knowledge, power and public trust

With some prescience, in 1995 the then newly appointed President of the General Medical Council (GMC), Sir Donald Irvine, observed: 'Self-regulation in any system – be it medicine or parliament – is built on trust. And if a gap grows between those who are regulating themselves and the public they serve – that's when the threat to self-regulation comes' (Smith, 1995: 1516). Three years later, the events at Bristol Royal Infirmary,

Table 1.1   Knowledge control and the politics of regulation

Arena of knowledge activity	Regulation functions		
	Standard setting	Monitoring and evaluation	Intervention
Creation (Research)	1	2	3
Transmission (Education)	4	5	6
Application (Performance)	7	8	9

that 'landmark in the history of self-regulation' as Klein describes it (Klein, 1998: 1741), converted a low-key public scepticism about medical authority into a high-profile, media-sensitive political issue of public trust, with the apparent momentum to refine the basis on which the profession relates to its erstwhile partners, civil society and the state.

Bristol achieved this because it focused attention on the profession's principal privilege and power: its unique access to, and control of, a body of knowledge that is highly valued by both civil society and state (Freidson, 1988). That control of knowledge both promotes and is dependent on public trust. Without it, the power of medicine and the triangle of political forces become obsolete. It is useful to view the control as being exercised through the three regulation functions of standards setting, monitoring and evaluation, and intervention, and applied to three arenas of knowledge activity: creation (research), transmission (teaching) and application (performance) (Table 1.1) (Salter, 1999: 149).

Each cell within the matrix constitutes a political territory over which competition for influence can occur: both within the medical profession, on the one hand, and between medicine, civil society and the state, on the other. There is no logical reason why public interest in the various facets of medical regulation should be restricted to one part of the matrix alone. In the UK, Bristol ensured that categories 7, 8 and 9 (doctor performance) attracted the initial media attention swiftly followed by categories 1, 2 and 3 following the revelations at Alder Hey concerning the absence of informed consent for the use of children's body parts in research. Equally, given the circumstances, the political debate could be further widened to include poorly trained and supervised junior doctors (categories 4, 5 and 6) – with a consequent impact on public trust.

Ultimately, any system of medical regulation rests on the twin powers of certification and licensing. In terms of Table 1.1, certification is a statement about the success or otherwise of the transmission of medical knowledge through education and, by its removal or limitation, can be used as a form of intervention (cell 6). Similarly, licensing, or registration, is a statement about the appropriate application of that knowledge in professional performance (fitness to practice) and can also be used as a form of intervention (cell 9). Ownership of these two powers is usually divided between several, or many, institutions which frequently do not integrate their regulatory activities. (Until recently, in the UK a doctor could be removed from the GMC's register yet retain his/her certification as a member or fellow of a Medical Royal College.) In addition, when under pressure to change, different institutions may produce different, and not necessarily compatible, responses couched in terms of one of the two powers without a clear understanding of their interrelationship. This then results in overlapping debates about re-certification, re-registration and revalidation.

Historically, the profession has demonstrated an ingenious capacity for evolving a plethora of institutions which engage in such competition for influence. When seen in terms of function, the internal organisation of medicine can be analysed in terms of five ideal types each of which make a particular functional contribution to the maintenance and enhancement of professional power: the learned society (preservation and advancement of the knowledge base), the certifying association (transmission and accreditation of knowledge), the licensing association (fitness to practice – knowledge application), the representative association (lobbying) and the trade union association (economic negotiation) (cf. Burrage *et al.*, 1990). In practice, of course, these ideal types will overlap and may be complemented by umbrella organisations which combine several functions. The first three types of institutions deal with the control of the knowledge resource itself and therefore constitute the institutional heart of clinical and professional autonomy. This autonomy enables the profession to negotiate with its economic and political environment in order to gain certain privileges as an occupational group in terms of pecuniary reward and political influence. If successful, these negotiations produce varying degrees of what may be termed economic autonomy (the ability to determine one's own system of economic rewards including market entry and exit) and political autonomy (the ability to determine the most important elements of health policy and its implementation), which constitute a surrounding set of defences against attempts by the state (or in some countries the market) to erode the fundamental professional autonomy (Elston, 1991).

Routine negotiations with the economic and political environments are usually conducted by a trade union or representative association which may be supported by, or merged with, one or more of the other four types. The tradition in the UK has been for the British Medical Association (BMA) to take the lead with the other organisations remaining discreetly in the background. Not so in other countries. In the Netherlands, for example, the Royal Dutch Society for the Promotion of Medicine (KNMG) is a federation of four medical associations including the National Association of Specialists (LSV) and the National Association of GPs (LHV) which not only acts as a trade union but also is responsible for the register of all qualified doctors, standards of professional conduct and medical ethics (Schepers and Casparie, 1997: 582). Clearly, such a concentration of functions increases the profession's bargaining power considerably. The trade union model is also dominant in Belgium though the function is divided between the Belgium Association of Medical Syndicates (BVAS) and the General Syndicate of Belgium Physicians (ASGB) which have different approaches to the economic and political environments. Whilst the BVAS holds true to the independent ethic of la médecine libérale the ASGB is quite willing to cooperate with the Health Insurance System and to form alliances with other groups. Thus, in 1975, it created a coalition with two smaller bodies to form the Confederation of Belgium Physicians and, where necessary, it links with the Federation of Belgium Associations of Medical Specialists (VBS) (Schepers, 1995).

Probably the most effective form of medical organisation for the negotiation of economic and political rewards exists in Germany where the Associations of Insurance Doctors combine the powers of compulsory membership with the control of market access. In order to treat patients covered by the sickness funds, doctors have to be members of one of the two Associations: the Verband der niederglasen Ärtze (representing doctors in independent local practice) and the Marburger Bund (representing salaried hospital doctors). Since these in turn have exclusive and legally sanctioned rights of negotiation with the sickness funds, the German medical profession's bargaining relationship with its economic environment is inherently favourable to its interests: that is, it has considerable economic autonomy (Moran and Wood, 1993: 61–5).

The extent to which the profession is able to negotiate effectively with economic and political pressures is dependent also on the institutional efficiency with which it regulates itself through the several control of knowledge functions (Table 1.1). In the UK, across the arenas of research, education and performance the standard setting activity has been undertaken by both learned societies (the specialist associations) and the certifying bodies (the universities and the Medical Royal Colleges); the monitoring largely by the Royal Colleges; and intervention by the latter (certification) and the GMC (licensing). However, with the move by the GMC towards the introduction of revalidation there is considerable pressure for these separate institutional contributions to form part of a single system rather than an uncoordinated set of informal arrangements. For the UK, this is sensitive and as yet uncharted political territory and international experience shows that even when procedural agreement is achieved this then has to be maintained. In the Netherlands, the KNMG's inclusion of regulatory, representation and negotiation functions presents an interesting case where, as Schepers and Casparie observe, 'a careful balancing act regarding self-regulation in a broader sense has to be performed with the KNMG and associated professional organisations' (Schepers and Casparie, 1997: 595). In the main the KNMG succeeds in maintaining its hold on the quality policies of the LSV, the LHV and the scientific societies but this is not always a straightforward process.

Division, rivalry and, on occasions, internecine conflict are more common features of the internal organisation of medicine than are harmony, sweetness and light. Given the breadth and complexity of the political territories summarised in Table 1.1 and the power inherent in their control, this is inevitable. Politics is after all a competitive business. Much of the competition is organised within and between the two arenas of education and performance which, institutionally, can be seen to be subject to the two powers of certification and licensing. Internationally, the established focus on education in the form of Continuing Medical Education (CME) and re-certification has often given the certifying institutions (mainly medical colleges rather than universities) the lead in the debate over how self-regulation can be improved. However, the certifying institutions are frequently dependent on individual specialist associations (learned societies) for the development of standards and this cooperation may not be forthcoming. For their part, specialist associations may decide that they are the appropriate bodies to regulate their members and view the medical colleges as distant and uninformed. Instances of such rivalry were common in the Netherlands in the 1980s among the organisations of both specialists and GPs as the profession began to respond to state pressure for quality assurance procedures to be introduced (Schepers and Casparie, 1997: 587).

The absence of a natural threshold between the concerns of certifying and licensing bodies means that their negotiating positions can be highly permeable. For example, those involved in the re-certification field have argued that the requirements of re-certification are more complex and technically demanding than those of certification and should include, as well as basic knowledge and competencies, a focus not only on non-clinical aspects of practice such as ethical conduct, interpersonal abilities and management skills but also, and more importantly, on job performance, process and outcomes (see e.g. Norcini, 1994; Southgate, 1994; Southgate and Jolly 1994). If this is the case, and fitness to practice is proven, the licensing body is left with nothing further to do but to issue the stamp of re-registration approval. In Canada, the national association of licensing authorities, the Federation of Medical Licensing Authorities of Canada, has resisted this implication and is establishing its own model for the maintenance and enhancement of professional performance (MEPP). Quite separately, the certifying bodies are continuing along their chosen route: the College of Family Physicians of Canada is commencing its maintenance of proficiency programme and the Royal College of Physicians and Surgeons of Canada its maintenance of competence programmes (Dauphinee, 1999). When or where the twain will meet is unknown. As the Canadian case illustrates, the dominance of institutional interest over what may be termed system functional efficiency can lead to the development of parallel and separate self-regulatory arrangements driven by equally insistent imperatives of territorial integrity.

Medicine and the state

At the macro-political level, the divisions within medicine are less important than the triangle of forces which promote the interdependence of profession and state. (The importance of the divisions re-emerges when that triangle is destabilised.) In his work on the health care state, Moran documents the mutual penetration that results from this interdependence:

> Professions are central to the life of the modern state: as concentrations of expertise; as sources of legitimising ideologies; as institutional apparatuses through which state power can be transmitted; and, more simply, as important pressure groups. Conversely, the modern state is central to the life of the professions. Professionalism is a strategy pursued to defend occupational interests, in involving the 'closure' of the occupation from market competition. That closure is typically enforced by authority drawn, in the last analysis, from the state. (Moran, 1999: 7)

In the case of the health care state, he suggests, the permanence of the symbiosis between the needs of the medical profession and those of the state has produced an alliance 'embedded' in democratic political arrangements and capitalist economic arrangements. Medicine and state form the core of a 'medical–industrial' complex linking corporate, professional and bureaucratic elites (Moran, 1999: chapter 6).

For both medicine and state, the most important political product of this arrangement is the ability of the profession to regulate the relationship between patient demand and health care supply. However configured, the terms of the orthodox medicine–state concordat give doctors a set of privileges which enable them to keep the patient in a subordinate market position. Thus in the UK, the profession extended the original principle of self-regulation of professional standards ceded in the 1858 Act to include the regulation of market entry and doctor supply (e.g. medical schools, the Medical Workforce Standing Advisory Committee), competitive conditions (e.g. the referral system, restrictions on advertising), market structures (e.g. designation by the Medical Practices Committee of the geographical distribution of general practice) and pay (the Review Body on Doctors and Dentists Remuneration, Merit Awards, the BMA's fee schedule for private practice) (Moran and Wood, 1993). By controlling the market for medical services and the nature of patients' interaction with it, the profession limits the extent to which patients can become active consumers capable of expressing an independent demand for health care. Rather, in the orthodox model, clinical and economic power overlap to ensure that, as far as possible, patient demand is defined with the orbit of medically defined patient 'need'.

The precise nature of the medicine–state relationship, and hence the particular foundation of long-term medical power, varies from country to country but in post-war Western Europe the 'medico-bureaucratic complex' became a common feature of government (Larkin, 1995: 45; see also Wohl, 1984). In the UK, it formed an integral part of the corporatist agreement accompanying the foundation of the NHS (Moran, 1995: 21–4). That agreement gave the profession power over the disposal of NHS resources, the ability 'to veto policy change by defining the limits of the acceptable and by determining the policy agenda', and confirmation of medicine's right to self-regulation (Day and Klein, 1992: 486). Over the succeeding decades the arrangement consolidated into a form of 'ideological corporatism' which ensured that policy was framed within a set of values acceptable to this particular knowledge elite to produce what some have characterised as the 'professionalised state' (Dunleavy, 1981; Dunleavy and O'Leary, 1987).

Other countries demonstrate a similar experience. In most cases it was the profession which in the early years dominated the corporatist arrangement in terms of discourse, structures and policy. An archetypal example is that of Norway where the legendary Dr Karl Evang became head of the Directorate of Health in 1938 and remained so for several decades, ably fusing the distinction between policy matters and those requiring medical competence (Erichsen, 1995a; see also Erichsen, 1995b). It was not until 1983 that a reorganisation separated the accountability lines of legal and medical expertise in government and not until 1992, that health policy became part of the policy mainstream with the appointment of the minister of health within the Ministry for Social Affairs. Since then the continuing decline of the medical hegemony in Norway and its ability to mould the health policy discourse has been evidenced by the redefinition of 'health policy experts' to mean health economists and social scientists rather than physicians. However, although in recognition of this decline the Norwegian

Medical Association has withdrawn from the formal policy formation arena, it continues to exercise considerable influence over
policy implementation (Erichsen, 1995a: 731).

Whilst the medicine–state relationship in Sweden and Spain
paralleled the Norway model in its immediate post-war form, a different, and as it was to prove less vulnerable, form of profession-
dominated corporatism developed in Germany, Belgium and the
Netherlands characterised by the inclusion of the sickness funds in
the corporatist arrangement. In health care politics, sickness funds
constitute a set of state-sanctioned institutions which through
their financial power have the potential to facilitate or resist
demands for change in the way medicine is governed. They can
create or oppose changes in the linkage between finance, on the
one hand, and the quantity and quality of care, on the other, and
any regulatory policy is obliged to work through them. In
Belgium, therefore, it is of some significance that the Technical
Medical Council of the Institut National d'Assurance Maladie-
Invalidité is composed entirely of doctors since it is the Council
which determines what medical acts with what relative weight
should be considered for reimbursement. This is reinforced by the
stipulation in the Law on the Practice of Medicine that the control
of key issues of medical practice lies with the Order of Physicians
(Schepers, 1995: 165).

At first sight, the situation in Germany is quite different with the
sickness funds Gesetzliche Krankenversicherung (GKV) administered by equal numbers of elected officials from associations of
employers and employees. This is deceptive because in practice the
funds have no authority to decide when and how the money is
spent. That decision is the result of negotiations between the
regional associations of sickness funds and the public law regional
associations of insurance doctors (Kassenärztliche Vereinigung –
KV). Since any physician who wishes to participate in the GKV is
required by law to be a member of a KV, which are administered
solely by physicians, the grip of the medical profession on the way
the sickness funds are used to implement policy is comprehensive
(Altenstetter, 1989: 160; Dohler, 1989: 184–5). KVs have a state
granted monopoly over the provision of health care, are legally
endowed with the right to self-governance (as are the sickness
funds), license their members for insurance practice, and take
corrective sanctions against their member doctors if their practice

patterns or charges exceed the norm (Giaimo, 1995: 360). And although the KVs are Länder (i.e. local state) based, this does not inhibit their ability to act in concert. As Freddi observes, 'When they [the KVs] negotiate economic transactions with the equally autonomous and corporatist sickness funds, or when they bargain with public authorities over annual increases of health expenditures, they act with one voice' – and their authority is cemented by the great normative power of legal forms typical of the German government tradition (Freddi, 1989: 14).

In countries where the sickness funds formed part of the medical profession's sphere of influence, the state for many years found itself colonised by the profession, rather than vice versa. Referring to the German case, Giaimo regards the concept of 'private interest government' as useful because it 'highlights the importance of delegated state authority, the crucial enforcement role of the state, and the ways that such a governance arrangement can allow the state to indirectly manage a policy area' such as health (Giaimo, 1995: 356). This is too one-sided a view and unjustifiably assumes a natural pre-eminence of the state in its relationship with medicine. Rather, it is clear that the profession's 'expert' dominance of the policy discourse can determine the state's policy agenda. Thus in the Federal Republic of Germany it was noted that professional preferences and diagnostic and therapeutic practices were respected by civil service hospital planners who supported medical progress. Bureaucrats and professionals were found to 'share similar values and perceptions about medicine and what is needed to practise it effectively and efficiently to the satisfaction of the public' (Altenstetter, 1989: 176).

France provides a sharp contrast to this picture of medical hegemony in the relationship between the state, sickness funds and the profession. Eighty per cent of the population are covered by the Caisse Nationale de l'Assurance Maladie des Travailleurs Salaries (CNAMTS) which governs a complex system of sixteen caisse régionales and 129 caisses locales. Most health policy is implemented through this national fund which fixes the levels of contribution, reimbursement, charges and fees. From the profession's perspective, the important part of this system is the 'convention': the standard fee schedule for all procedures and consultations (Wilsford, 1991: 125). Given France's political culture of centralised étatisme, it is not surprising to learn that the state uses the periodic renegotiation of the convention as a means for imposing its will on the doctors – so much so that one commentator has described French medicine as 'administered medicine' (Freddi, 1989: 17). Be that as it may, what is clear is that the ability of medicine to resist the imperatives of the state are diminished by its lack of influence over the sickness funds and, as a result, its fragmented internal organisation becomes particularly exposed.

In Europe, the professions emerged before the fully fledged nation state and so were in position to attempt to negotiate a mutually acceptable political bargain to deal with the growth in citizenship welfare rights. However, where the consolidation of the state occurred first, medicine has found itself in a weak and marginal position, unable to penetrate the state apparatus. Thus in Mexico the corporatist arrangement between the state and the ruling political party ensured that social benefits were delivered through the party political organisations to which the medical profession, along with other social groups, was subordinate. With no real power base, the profession was obliged to accept a state-imposed system of medical regulation where, in company with other professions, medicine was subject to the 1944 Law of the Professions. This gave the state the prerogative to establish licensing procedures which explicitly excluded professional groups from the decision-making process. Even within the health delivery system, doctors fared little better. Although they secured the middle managerial positions in the Instituto Mexicano del Seguro Social (IMSS – 70 per cent of whose budget was allocated to health), they remained politically peripheral and, as Nigenda observes, 'could not define the institution's internal policy, influence the recruitment of personnel, or negotiate their own contractual and salary conditions' (Nigenda, 1997: 87).

Corporatism (of whatever kind) is, of course, by no means a universal feature of the medicine–state relationship. To the political culture of the USA, such an arrangement is anathema and an offence against the traditions of institutional pluralism and government by contract. Medicine and its regulatory institutions remain determinedly separate from the state, but as the American Medical Association (AMA) bears witness, no less powerful for that. For decades, it was able to use its lobbying muscle to thwart attempts to introduce a national health insurance scheme and only accepted the introduction of the Medicare/Medicaid bill in 1965 on condition that the profession would continue to charge fees – that is, maintain its economic autonomy. It could perhaps be argued that the state licensing boards in the US constitute examples of the medical profession combining with 'the local state' to regulate doctors, though the extreme variations in the disciplinary activities of different state licensing boards, the differences in state laws, and the lack of coordinating machinery between state boards considerably diminish the significance of this particular political union (Moran and Wood, 1993: 76). Of rather more significance are the professional monitoring measures which formed part of the original state funded Medicare and Medicaid programmes, not because they became an instrument of the state will but because they were eventually to metamorphose into Utilisation Review used by the market-based Health Maintenance Organisations (HMOs) (Björkman, 1989: 51–4). Not that this was in any sense a development deliberately fostered by an alliance between the state and the health care industry. For just as the anti-corporatist instincts of American political culture militate against a state–medicine union, so also are they opposed to the public elision of state–industry interests.

The power relations embedded in the medicine–state relationship determine both the nature of medical self-regulation and the possible responses to the demands for change. Given the variety of forms that relationship can assume in terms of the proximity of the partners, their legal and institutional connections, the degree of ideological overlap in their policy discourse, and the balance of power between them it is inevitable that the national arrangements for the governance of medicine should, as expressions and measures of the relationship, faithfully reflect this diversity. There is, as Moran and Wood observe, what is best described as a continuum of medical governance rather than a set of distinctive types (Moran and Wood, 1993: 91–3). That continuum ranges from entirely government institutions in terms of legal status, procedures and membership, through state-sponsored but professionally controlled bodies, to totally independent professional entities. Furthermore, it should be understood that regulation is not necessarily a one-way process but an integral part of the balance of power between medicine and state. Such has been the interdependence of medicine and state that in some cases it has been the former which has regulated the latter, for example, through a decisive influence over health policy, rather than vice versa. The implication of this analysis is that we can expect the response to the demands for change to be equally diverse. Differences in the juxtapositioning of formative political forces in the medicine–state relationship are bound to produce a differentiated set of responses.

Reformulating the concordat

The quantity and quality of the clinical care provided in any system of health care is determined by doctors' decisions. Other factors such as resource availability may constrain or facilitate those decisions, but it is doctors who through their diagnostic and therapeutic judgements determine the pattern of clinical care and it is the structure of medical regulation which most intimately governs their behaviour. When, as appears to be a universal process, citizens demand more and better health care, the state must respond and attempt to readjust the demand–supply mismatch. Almost invariably, and unless the medical profession is able to anticipate the demands of citizens, that response includes seeking to change the behaviour of doctors in order to control the cost implications of the increased demand. This, in turn, frequently means that the regulatory procedures of medicine must be reformulated accordingly and, given that these form part of the profession's system of self-government, so also must the state's concordat with the profession.

Where a corporatist arrangement exists, the most radical solution is for the state to abandon its alliance with medicine, seek to impose its own definition of how health care should be supplied and re-shape the context in which doctors work. No longer perceived as politically functional, the profession is then excluded from its privileged position in policy making. The UK's experience with the emergence of the internal market policy in 1989–90 where the profession found itself comprehensively cold-shouldered is one example of this. A rather more substantial example in terms of a lasting loss of medical power, is that of Italy. Here the sickness funds, the *casse mutue*, with which the profession was heavily identified, proved unable to cope with rising demand and were duly removed by the 1978 reform which introduced a single unitary scheme covering all citizens, the Servizio Sanitario Nazionale (SSN). At the same time, broad political shifts, including the strengthening of the left (particularly the Communist Party (PCI)) and the establish-ment of powerful regions decimated the traditional power of the profession, severed its links with policy making and drastically reduced the significance of its remaining rights of self-regulation (Ferrera, 1989: 126). Over-reliance on a corporatism based on an alliance with a single party, the Christian Democrats, had cost the profession dear.

In other parts of Europe, the traditional corporatism has been redefined in a less dramatic fashion as the state has attempted to bring the profession to heel in the interests of cost-containment. In so doing, it has used a combination of legal and economic measures to try to alter the context in which medical practice takes place with a consequent impact on the freedoms of self-regulation. In Belgium, the 1993 Law Moureaux on health and disability gave more power to employers, trade unions and government over the finances of the health care system in terms of the setting of both global budgets and those of specific sectors. However, the difficulty the state then faced was enforcing this policy through the complex array of sickness funds where doctors held consider-able sway as part of the original concordat (Schepers, 1995: 171). As is customary in its dealings with the medical profession, the state found policy formation easier than policy implementation.

A rather more specific legal impact was achieved in Sweden where the 1970 Seven Crowns Reform removed the right of doctors to their own financial transactions with patients and established the machinery for national salary negotiations as a vehicle for the con-trol of doctors' incomes and hence of costs. In formal terms, med-ical power was further reduced by the 1982 Health and Sick Care Law which removed the previous legal stipulation that the head of a clinic had to be a physician thus apparently opening the door for the rise of managerial power. This was accompanied by the setting up of a central agency, the Health and Medical Services Disciplinary Board, to deal with patients' complaints against doctors (the pro-cedure was known as the Lex Maria) – seemingly a recognition of patient power. Devolution of the health service to the county councils added further to the sense of an end to the old corporate alliance between medicine and state. Although that alliance has been substantially redefined, clinical autonomy as embodied in the procedures of self-regulation has not been seriously challenged. Managers and patients have not taken over. This may be because, as Dohler argues, for the state cost-containment was the key issue and 'a reduction of professional autonomy could be avoided best if physicians were able to restrain, or at least postpone, their economic demands' (Dohler, 1989: 196). If the state can solve the problem of excess citizen demand by restricting supply and cost without confronting the issue of medical self-governance then it will do so. That way professional autonomy is respected, part of the concordat can be retained and with it the benefits of the covert rationing function.

As the state moves to deal with the cost implications of increased demand, so the profession's involvement with different types of payment systems becomes an increasingly important factor in the political game and a measure of its ability to protect clinical autonomy, or not, as the case may be. In France, the state's dominance of the sickness funds and periodic manipulation of the 'convention', the standard fee schedule, gave it the means to insist that doctors should implement the policy of 'le bon usage des soins' (the wise use of health care services) introduced in 1986. Under the Plan Séguin some illnesses were exonerated from co-payments. To be successful, the Plan required doctors to discriminate clearly between exonerated and non-exonerated illnesses. In return for implementing a policy which reduced patients' rights by eliminating reimbursement or introducing charges, they received a fee increase (Wilsford, 1991: 148–9). Control of fees was also an initial plank of the Canadian state's strategy to increase its regulation of the profession and, once established, signalled the beginning of a decline in medical power (Coburn, 1993: 844). Even in the USA, that most pluralistic of societies, from 1992 the Medicare payments were based on fee schedules derived from the Resource Based Relative Value Scales (RBRVS).

From the impartial perspective of the economist, it has been argued that 'licensing is sought by doctors because it can be used to reduce supply and thereby lessen competition and enhance income' (Moran and Wood, 1993: 35). Pursuing the same logic, if the state can increase the supply of doctors then greater competition will produce a reduction in income (and health care costs) as a way of responding to increased citizen demand. Part of the French state's strategy was to achieve precisely this. That it was able to expand the supply of doctors from the mid-1960s onwards was because the state, rather than the profession, regulates French medical education and the number of students admitted (Wilsford, 1991: 128). Similarly, in Canada the state is now directly involved in medical education and the supply of doctors through its control over university and hospital funding, internships and residency places (Coburn, 1993: 844). Therefore, to achieve the economic and political manipulation of doctor supply, and *pace* Moran and Wood, it is more important for the state to regulate education than licensing. In addition, in the French case the absence of a referral system and a GP gatekeeping function reduces the ability of the French medical profession to resist the competitive pressures fostered by the state because patient choice is widened rather than narrowly directed through a series of professionally controlled access points.

In contrast to France and Canada, the capacity of the German state to use the economy of health care to redirect doctor behaviour and so redefine its concordat with medicine is restricted by the close relationship between the profession and the sickness funds. In the wake of what was widely perceived to be a cost explosion in health care, the 1988 Health Care Reform Act and the 1992 Health Care Structural Reform Act were introduced with the aim of stabilising insurance contributions by capping medical and prescription budgets. Doctors' associations played little part in the formulation of the policy and indeed opposed it at many points: an indication that the corporatism of yesteryear was no more. However, as others have discovered elsewhere, although the state could place the profession on the margins of policy formation, policy implementation is dependent upon the power structures at the local level of the health service, the Länder, where medicine still ruled as it always had done. As a result, despite government threats concerning state intervention in substantive areas of self-regulation in the event of professional non-compliance in policy implementation, the details of its enactment remained a matter for the KVs and the sickness funds. KVs became responsible for cost overruns and the monitoring of their members' practice which merely served to emphasise the state's dependence on the profession (Giaimo, 1995: 363–6). In this important sense nothing had changed despite the rhetoric of the state. Private interest government is alive and well.

As the French case demonstrates, control of the economy of health care removes the need for direct intervention in medical regulation and the internal affairs of the profession because the redirection of doctor behaviour to deal with rising costs, the object of the exercise, is achieved by economic means. Conversely, in Germany the inability to control that economy without the cooperation of doctors' associations has revealed the limits of state power: an alternative reason for leaving medical self-regulation alone. However, a different scenario emerges and different pressures on the medicine–state concordat are generated when the state is concerned to respond to citizen demands for better, as well as more, health care.

In the Netherlands, the state used the sickness funds to place pressure on the medical profession to introduce quality assurance procedures. Prompted by government moves in the mid-1970s encouraging the sickness funds to introduce the external audit of doctors, the National Organisation for Quality Assurance was established by the LSV and the Association of Medical Hospital Directors as a professional defence against the potential intrusions of government, health insurers and hospital managers (Schepers and Casparie, 1997: 585). As a tactic this obviously succeeded because it was not until the late 1980s that a resurgent demand from the state for a national quality care policy culminating in three national conferences produced agreement that the primary responsibility for the quality of care lay with the providers.

Interestingly, the interpretation of this policy is that the focus of the external review by insurers and patients should be the measures taken to assure the provision of high quality care and not the quality of the care itself: in other words, process and not outcomes. As Schepers and Casparie observe, what this meant was that 'the leading role of the medical profession in the development of medical quality assurance was acknowledged by other actors in Dutch health care' (Schepers and Casparie, 1997: 585). Medical self-regulation remained intact. This dependence posed serious problems for the process of policy implementation. It was not until 1996 that agreement between the factions of Dutch medicine was reached thus enabling the introduction of a law on the re-registration of all medical practitioners every five years.

The course adopted by the Dutch state in responding to citizen demands for better quality clinical care is a common one. Where self-regulation forms part of the corporatist arrangement, the state has first placed pressure on the profession and then waited for its internal politics to produce a solution – with varying degrees of success depending on the extent of professional divisions. In Belgium, the state reconfirmed the therapeutic freedom of doctors in its 1989 Programme-Law but at the same time introduced the new legal obligation for doctors 'to refrain from prescribing unnecessary, expensive investigations and treatment and from carrying out or having carried out unnecessary treatment at the expense of the obligatory Health Insurance System' (Schepers, 1995: 173): symbolically impressive but meaningless in practical terms unless mechanisms could then be developed to implement such good intentions. Since this required the cooperation of the profession, it has taken some time. In 1993 BVAS and the sickness funds reached agreement on the accreditation of medical practitioners at set intervals based on criteria developed by doctors regarding activities such as the keeping of medical records, a stipulated amount of continuing medical education, and participation in quality assurance activities; the whole process to be supported by local peer review groups.

It is an interesting reflection on medical power, and the state's need to acknowledge it, that the approach to re-accreditation adopted in the Belgium case should have consistent international parallels elsewhere. Where the quality of clinical care is at issue, the regulatory methods adopted have in the main followed the contours of medicine's institutions and culture in ways which, first, exclude non-professionals from the standard setting, evaluation and intervention activities and, second, focus on matters of educational process rather than performance outcomes. The concordat between medicine and state may be redefined, but its recognition of the profession's control of medical knowledge (its essential power) remains intact.

Hence in the Netherlands, the law allows for two methods of re-registration: working in a practice that is evaluated by peers and coordinated by the Dutch Association of Medical Specialists, or fulfilling the continuing medical education requirements of the specialist societies (Swinkels, 1999: 1191). Similarly, the maintenance of professional standards programmes run by the Australian and New Zealand medical colleges are based on collecting points for CME and quality assurance activities and most do not have practice-based components (Newble *et al.*, 1999: 1185). Nor, unlike the Belgium and Dutch examples, are they mandatory – with the exception of the Royal Australian College of Obstetricians and Gynaecologists which has a true re-certification procedure in that there is a three-year time limit applied to the award of its fellowship diploma. Whether the programmes will remain a voluntary professional activity outside the purview of the Australian state for much longer is questionable despite their 'being sold to the membership as a pre-emptive strike against revalidation procedures being imposed from outside' (Newble *et al.*, 1999: 1186). Most states may accept the inevitability of self-regulation but they are under increasing pressure to make the maintenance of standards through re-registration or re-certification a legal requirement rather than a matter of professional judgement. The question is at what point they do so. Making the requirement a statutory duty before the profession has established the internal procedures for implementation risks policy failure and political exposure to the demands of public opinion. However, not making it a statutory duty risks allowing the profession to continue to engage in expert obfuscation. It is clearly a difficult tension to handle, which is why France, Germany and Switzerland, for example, have yet to take the legal plunge.

For the most part, in countries where there is a tradition of professional self-regulation resulting from a corporate relationship between medicine and the state, the demand from citizens for improvements in the quality of clinical care has been met with procedures which concentrate on the education of the doctor rather than on his/her performance. In terms of the requirements of individual professional autonomy, this emphasis is understandable because it does not question the doctor's application of medical knowledge (i.e. performance) but measures whether that knowledge base is appropriately updated, a less intrusive procedure, and so forms part of categories 4, 5 and 6 of Table 1.1 rather than categories 7, 8 and 9. In terms of the requirements of public trust, it will almost certainly prove to be inadequate. In contrast to this, in countries where a medicine–state concordat has never existed, or is very weak, and where the private sector is the dominant player in health care provision, the profession can be forced to accept that its control of its knowledge base is neither unique nor sacrosanct.

In the USA, the introduction by government in 1982 of diagnostic related groups (DRGs) – clinical procedure categories with a fixed price for each – as part of the Medicare programme provided the platform for the development of procedures, external to the profession, for the regulation of performance. This process was facilitated by a state organisation, the Health Care Finance Administration (HCFA), which issued contracts to peer review organisations for the conduct of quality control and utilisation review activities based on DRGs. As the commercial pressures of cost-containment increased, hospital administrators and purchasing agencies took advantage of the HCFA's procedures to introduce controls over medical decision making. Judgements about the use of medical knowledge were no longer the special province of doctors alone and, as Björkman observes, an 'outstanding aspect of the DRG programme [was] the transfer of power by Congress from physician and hospital providers to the federal bureaucracy' (Björkman, 1989: 60). In a market driven economy of managed health care, the question facing the purchasers is straightforward: 'Should [they] write reimbursement cheques for whatever the doctor orders or does an insurer have the right to evaluate the appropriateness of the treatment before paying for it?' (Ross, 1999: 616).

As in other countries, in the US the medical profession has taken steps to regulate the standard of its members' performance but this has remained a separate exercise from the quality control activities of the health care market and has not restricted the latter's incursions into professional territory. Of the 24 boards that are members of the American Board of Medical Specialties all have limited, or plan to limit, the duration of validity of their certificates to between seven and ten years. In the main, their re-certification procedures are based on CME or examinations (Norcini, 1994, 1999; Norcini and Dawson-Saunders, 1994; Norcini and Shea, 1997).

Conclusions

The international evidence supports the theoretical proposition that the manner in which citizen rights and demand for more and better health care are translated into new policies is dependent, in the first instance, on the state's willingness and ability to redefine its relationship with the profession and so alter the balance of the triangle of forces between itself, medicine and civil society. Where there has been a corporate relationship, the state has universally moved to create distance between itself and the profession, to diminish medicine's influence over policy making and to increase its own ability to manage the demand–supply mismatch. Control of the economic context of medical decision making is a key factor in what happens next. Where the state has that control, as in France, the economic autonomy of the profession, its first line of defence, is reduced and it is obliged to respond to state pressures. Where the profession retains control, as in Germany, it may respond to state pressures but on its own terms. Direct state intervention in the regulatory affairs of the profession is rare, not least because the state is wisely hesitant about assuming responsibility for the quality of care. However, where the state has given the private sector a prominent role in the delivery of health care, as in the USA, commercial considerations have overridden any qualms about such intervention.

For the most part, the changes in the corporatist arrangement can be described as a 'rebalancing' of that arrangement rather than its elimination; not, as Giaimo has argued, as a strategic government act but as a natural consequence of the interdependence of medicine and state (Giaimo, 1995: 368). As Moran and Wood point out, even where a state wishes to exercise more control over the medical profession it cannot always do so: there is 'an implementation gap' between policy goals and their enactment derived from the fact that doctors' 'greatest influence lies less in their overt intervention in politics, and more in the way their everyday influence in regulation shapes outcomes' (Moran and Wood, 1993: 136). Thus, for example, the profession may have accepted the policy goal that reform of its self-regulation of standards is necessary, but its implementation of that goal has generally been expressed in terms of the monitoring of continuing education (an unconvincing proxy) rather than performance though this is now beginning to change as the need for public reassurance becomes greater.

In general theoretical terms, the British case reflects the international experience though perhaps in more intensified form. The macro-level engagement between medicine, civil society and the state and the pervasive implications of that engagement for other levels of medical politics is a dominating force. As a consequence of the dynamic of health care rights embodied within British citizenship, civil society places political demands upon the state which are ever-increasing, always refining and never retreating.

Citizens expect that there will always be more and better health care. At the same time, the expansion of tax-based revenues for the NHS has never been sufficient to meet civil society demand. There has always been a mismatch of demand and supply. In reflecting on how to respond, the state's political imagination is restricted to options acceptable to the hegemony of the welfare state ideology which rejects values on which an appeal for citizen rights to be stabilised or reduced might be based. The experience of Thatcherism was that its supposed attack on welfare rights resulted not in a diminishment of rights but in a consumerist redefinition of how the state should deliver those rights.

If the state is thus unable explicitly to manage the demand side of the political equation, it has three choices: it can attempt a qualitative shift in the increase of supply side resources, it can seek a more efficient management of supply or it can search for a form of covert rationing. The former two have been tried at various times. They have never worked because in the absence of any cost to the health consumer the demand for health care is highly, if not perfectly, elastic. This then leaves the option of rationing by those who dispose of health care resources to patients: the doctors. In order to carry out this system function, doctors must retain their authority, legitimacy and the trust of patients in the way in which they create, transmit and apply medical knowledge. For this reason, and as with all countries, the self-regulation of the profession is the policy touchstone of the politics of medicine because its purpose is to sustain the relationship between both medicine and civil society, on the one hand, and medicine and the state, on the other.

Analysing medical regulation in terms of the knowledge control functions of standard setting, monitoring and evaluation, and intervention demonstrates the range of political territories which have to be addressed in exploring the politics of medicine (Table 1.1). The evolving relationship between medicine, civil society and the state produces demands for change which may require a response in any or all of these territories. Yet the very stability of the concordat between medicine and state in the UK militates against an efficient response from the many institutions of the profession because they have, until recently, slept the sleep of the just, largely undisturbed by the vicissitudes of the outside political world. When the Merrison Committee on the regulation of the medical profession reported in 1975, it was doing so as the first inquiry since the original ceding of self-regulatory powers by the state in the 1858 Medical Act. Consequently, and historically, in the absence of any external pressure for organisational rationality, the profession has produced a kaleidoscope of institutional solutions to regulatory issues which accommodated its many and varied internal interests. Diversity, not efficiency, has been the watchword. Nor are the internal differences between medical institutions conducive to amicable political intercourse when regulatory territory is at stake.

The traditional inertia of the medicine's institutions was a product of the long-standing marriage between the profession and the state. Sustained by the triangle of forces, both felt comfortable in an arrangement where the state for decades acted protectively towards its spouse, believing that it was in its own interest and that of civil society to allow medicine the freedom it desired. Unlike other countries, the UK's situation was not complicated by the presence of sickness funds with their capacity to add an extra, and possibly disturbing, dimension to the medicine–state relationship. Elite assumptions and negotiations could therefore be simplified and agreements more easily reached. Policy making took place within routinised procedures where the parameters of acceptable policies were well established and trade-offs a part of normal custom and practice.

It is within this framework that the pressures, events and policies described in this book must be seen. With the developments at Bristol, Alder Hey and elsewhere, the civil society dimension of the triangle of forces has been activated to an unprecedented degree. Sustained media involvement has contributed to a highly visible politicisation of the medicine–state concordat which is likely to be an enduring feature of the future of the politics of medicine. The balance of power within the triangle of forces has, it would seem, shifted as the profession's institutions have vibrated in the political heat. But does this mean that the systemic significance of medicine is therefore diminished, or that the dependence of the state on the profession's ability to handle the demand–supply conundrum is any less? As the international evidence demonstrates, reformulation of a relationship is not necessarily the same as a redistribution of power. In this respect, continuity is at least as possible as change.

2

The politics of the doctor–patient relationship

Introduction

The relationship between doctors and patients is at the heart of medical power. Within its compass are negotiated the micro-politics of expert knowledge, the authority of professional values and the allocation of health care resources. From the many aspects of its nature flow the singular significance of public trust in medicine, the necessity of the edifice of self-regulation and, indeed, the very basis of the concordat between medicine and the state. For these reasons the relationship deserves close scrutiny. The purpose of this chapter is to examine the different understandings of its complex dimensions, to identify the ways in which power operates within the confines of the relationship, and thus to determine the implications of this micro-engagement between civil society and medicine for the macro-level of politics.

First, there is the issue of how the traditional relationship between doctors and patients has been understood. To what extent do those understandings provide us with a useful analytical grip on the politics of the relationship and the micro-power of doctors? Second, what are the perceived challenges to that traditional relationship, what evidence exists to substantiate them and how are they seen to have emerged? Third, how can we reconcile the different views of the relationship? Is the medical professional a politically reflexive animal or is his response to challenge constrained by an overwhelming sense of cultural self-worth?

The traditional doctor–patient relationship

There are as many orthodoxies in social science as there are in medicine and it is interesting to see how over time these have evolved a variety of analyses of the doctor–patient relationship, some more illuminating than others. In part, this has been in response to changes in the empirical reality of doctor–patient relations but in part also, one suspects, as a consequence of epistemic conflicts within social science itself. In other words, social science is not an impartial arbiter of the world of doctor and patient but a politically engaged participant in it.

In its early days, the understanding of the traditional doctor–patient relationship was based on a straightforward paternalistic model. Here the doctor has exclusive control over the definition and dispensation of relevant medical knowledge regarding diagnosis and therapy and the patient accepts both the authority of the doctor to exercise this control and the consequent legitimacy of his decisions. Doctors are active and patients are passive: a perfectly balanced power relationship. Talcott Parsons provides an early example of this model in his conceptualisation of the sick role. Doctors are seen as controlling the role in terms of both its rights and its obligations. Thus by being designated as 'sick', patients are excused other role-related activities such as those of family and work but on condition that they accept the obligation to try to get well, seek expert help and comply with the medical regimen (Parsons, 1951).

The concept of the subordinate sick role resonates easily with other work on the asymmetry of doctor and patient knowledge and in particular on the privileging of expert over lay knowledge and perspectives. Both point to the inevitability of doctor dominance. Richard Titmuss helped consolidate the sociological view of patient subordination when he argued that consumers of health care are in a uniquely vulnerable position because they are unable to determine how much medical care they need, are poorly equipped to assess the value of the care they receive and are heavily reliant on doctors' advice and expertise (Titmuss, 1968). Similarly, in their application of economic theory to the doctor–patient relationship, health economists describe it as an 'agency relationship' between professionals and the consumers of health care (Shackley and Ryan, 1994). Such agency relationships are characterised by an asymmetry of information between a principal (an uninformed player) and an agent (an informed player) who acts on behalf of the principal. The extra twist in the case of health care, and the unusual dimension of medical power, is that the consumers' agents (the doctors) are also the suppliers of health care. As a consequence, and unlike other market situations, the utility functions of doctor and patient are no longer independent but interdependent: the provider has interests which are partly congruent and partly in conflict with those of the patient.

The political significance of the simple dichotomy between those who have knowledge and those who do not is reinforced if one accepts the view that the social construction of 'facts', and what is regarded as valuable facts, is in general biased towards expert knowledge at the expense of lay knowledge (Jasanoff and Wynne, 1998). Experts are seen to provide knowledge and lay people, to use it as part of a natural social process. Thus, in the clinical environment, the privileged status of the doctor's expert knowledge is naturally dominant over any lay knowledge the patient may bring to the encounter. Patients, it is argued, are obliged to act within the medical knowledge domain (Falkum and Førde, 2001; Roberts and Aruguete, 2000).

Explanations of how doctors maintain the asymmetry of knowledge between themselves and patients, invoke their status as experts and thus retain control of their primary political territory, tend to focus on the nature of the discourse within that arena. Doctors are seen as not simply imposing their expert biomedical view of the world on grateful patients but as using a variety of communicative techniques to achieve agreement on their terms. For example, clinicians may include the patient's perspective but only after the diagnosis has been given and an agreed framework of understanding established. They may disregard some patient questions, reposition others, delay answering or not answer at all and, if necessary, re-invoke the explicit clinical agenda to regain control of the medical encounter (see e.g. Gill, 1998; Roberts, 2000).

Just as social scientists have developed a critique based on the many and varied ways in which doctors manipulate the interaction with their patients, so large numbers of medical scientists have explored the same territory and created a considerable literature with the objective of understanding how patient 'compliance' with a given medical regimen can be more efficiently achieved (Trostle, 1988). As Talcott Parsons would probably have agreed, non-compliant patients can be presented as a problem for the medical profession because they do not observe the obligations of the patient role to adhere to medical advice – from a traditional standpoint, the *sine qua non* of effective treatment. At its most coercive, the compliance literature teaches physicians how to manipulate their patients' behaviour without questioning their own beliefs, without increasing their patients' understanding or without being found out (Benfari *et al.*, 1981; Rodin and Janis, 1979). It is an impressive, if unreflective, accolade to the principle of the dominant doctor. It is also, as Trostle observes, 'an ideology that transforms physicians' theories about the proper behaviour of patients into a series of research strategies, research results, and potentially coercive interventions that *appear* appropriate, and that reinforce physicians' authority over health care' (Trostle, 1988: 1300, his emphasis).

As such it can be argued that it forms part of an established medical ideology which insists that any apparent conflict between doctor and patient interests can readily be resolved by the doctor because, first, doctors always act in the interests of their patients provided they are given the clinical freedom to do so and, second, patients are not in a position to determine their own health care needs accurately. Even if patients could acquire relevant information they would, it is suggested, lack the expertise to interpret it in the light of their own interests. The neatness of the political equation (doctors' interests equal patients' interests) leads into a supporting set of values concerning the need to protect its finely balanced mathematics from the possible distorting effect of the market. Any influence which could persuade either doctors or patients that their interests are in fact different is to be resisted and, if possible, eliminated. Hence, professional control of the environment in which doctors and patients interact, such as market controls, becomes both necessary, justifiable and a natural consequence of the traditional patient–doctor relationship.

In her seminal work on the GMC, Meg Stacey quotes an example of these values at work in the response of the GMC to the Monopolies and Mergers Commission's (MMC) inquiry in 1988–89 into the long established restrictions on advertising by doctors. Promotional advertising should be opposed in the public interest, the Council maintained, because it would exploit the ignorance and vulnerability of sick and mentally ill patients and would reduce the trust between doctor and patient by implying that some doctors were not fully competent (Stacey, 1992a: 191–4). As Stacey observes, this response 'exhibits distrust of patients' satisfaction with treatment as a reliable indicator of the quality of service' (Stacey, 1992a: 192). It assumes not only that patients cannot determine what they want, but also that they cannot evaluate what they get. In support of the GMC's position, a *British Medical Journal* leader argued that the MMC had failed to understand the nature of the doctor–patient relationship where self-promotional advertising is inconsistent with the philosophy of a caring profession (Havard, 1989; quoted by Stacey, 1992a: 193). The relationship had to be protected from such undesirable influences.

If the studies of the patient–doctor relationship portray it as characterised by asymmetric knowledge, privileged experts, techniques of communicative dominance and an overarching set of values which legitimate doctor dominance, then, in terms of general social trends, the medicalisation thesis would appear to be the natural consequence of these findings. This is the argument that the jurisdiction of medicine is constantly expanding to include new problems within its definition of 'normality' and the proper functioning, deportment and control of the human body (see e.g. Lupton, 1994; Zola, 1972). As the medical scientific knowledge base expands, it is contended, so medicine is able to bring new behaviours within the orbit of professional surveillance by defining them as medical, rather than social conditions (e.g. various forms of social deviancy such as alcoholism and drug addiction) (Conrad and Schneider, 1985). Thus the province where this new knowledge is applied, that of the patient–doctor relationship, becomes ever more varied as the new conditions become part of the consulting room agenda. At the same time, medicine's very ability to reinvent itself as an agent of new forms of social control acts to reinforce its social legitimacy and social power. There is considerable resonance between the medicalisation thesis and the Foucauldian view of medicine as part of a wider, more extensive apparatus of surveillance concerned with the moral regulation and 'normalisation' of the population (Foucault, 1973). Here there is an emphasis on the exercise of disciplinary power which through the 'clinical gaze' reduces the body to something 'docile' that can be 'surveilled, used, transformed and improved'. As with the medicalisation thesis, the assumption is that medical power is pervasive, that the sites of opposition are few and that the dynamic is irreversible.

The cumulative effect of these understandings of the context and nature of the doctor–patient relationship is to suggest the theoretical and empirical inevitability of medical dominance. The patient is passive, manipulated or seduced, the micro-politics stable and the future predictable. Little room is left for the possibility of conflict. Medical power, it would seem, is implacable and unproblematic.

The challenge

A number of approaches and studies have converged to challenge this deterministic and static interpretation of the doctor–patient relationship. In part they can be seen as a reaction against the well worn but unimaginative dimensions of the previous analyses, in part the introduction of new evidence and sources of evidence, and in part the dim realisation that life could not possibly be that simple. Certainly, it is not just a case of social scientists redrawing their understandings in response to changes in the external world but rather that, as part of that world, they have also changed. From an ordered perspective of a world of medical hegemony, regrettable but explicable according to established sociological tenets of medical power, the view has shifted to one of a world of uncertainty where the dimensions of professional control are much less easy to identify.

Central to this view is a reassessment of the role of knowledge in human relations and the much reduced ability of any single group consistently to order, control and dispense a particular body of knowledge to its political advantage. Giddens's influential work on 'late' modernity argues that the constant production and dissemination of new knowledge creates a situation where beliefs and practices are subject to regular examination, scrutiny and revision. As a result, what he terms 'reflexivity' becomes a chronic and defining feature of society, replacing the old stabilities of traditional social relations with the 'manufactured uncertainty' of late modernity (Giddens, 1991, 1994). Expert systems are destabilised and with them the old ways of legitimating power through the authoritative distribution of scientific knowledge. As Williams and Calnan observe, for social relations this means that 'contexts of actions become pluralised and a diversity of authorities and expertise exist for the charting, planning and organisation of modern social life ... lay views towards science and technology, including modern medicine, come to comprise a shifting dialectic of trust and doubt, certainty and uncertainty, reverence and disillusionment' (Williams and Calnan, 1996: 1613). Public trust in medicine, that key indicator of medical authority in the doctor–patient relationship, can no longer be assumed but has to be actively negotiated, won and retained. Once gained it can, Giddens maintains, still be lost because 'attitudes of trust, as well as more pragmatic acceptance, scepticism, rejection and withdrawal, uneasily coexist in the social space linking individual activities and expert systems' (Giddens, 1991: 7). In making this claim, Giddens echoed the themes already promulgated by the advocates of the 'deprofessionalisation' thesis that the cultural authority of medicine is in decline (Haug, 1973, 1988; Starr, 1982), but placed them in a much broader context of knowledge-driven social change.

Giddens's claims regarding the permeability and vulnerability of expert systems have been reinforced by Ulrich Beck's analysis regarding the social risks that these systems both produce and seek to regulate. This suggests that as science continues to drive the process of change in modern society, so it creates risks in terms of, for example, environmental pollution or human disease; moreover, risks which are increasingly unacceptable to the cultural beliefs of society. If science, including medical science, were able to use its traditional authority to persuade citizens that these risks could be adequately regulated then the political problem would be avoided. However, Beck's argument is that 'the history of the growing consciousness and social recognition of risks coincides with the history of the demystification of science' (Beck, 1992: 59). Science and scientists, therefore, are politically exposed.

Their exposure and discomfort is magnified, some have argued, not only because their knowledge boundaries are permeable but also because citizens have found ways of establishing their own knowledge base in opposition to that of science. As a consequence, the old reliance of doctors on an asymmetric knowledge relationship with their patients as the basis for their interpersonal power has been undermined. In his theory of communicative action, Habermas suggests that people have developed the means and the confidence to recognise the importance of their own 'life worlds' as a source of expertise which they can bring to bear on particular problems hitherto colonised by the rational discourse of science (Habermas, 1985). Thus in the case of medicine, self-help groups have enabled citizens with particular diseases or conditions to value their own life worlds and to regard their moral and practical understandings of their situation as a legitimate part of any discourse about appropriate therapy (Kelleher, 1994). Within the supporting social framework of the self-help group, experiential knowledge becomes the vehicle for understanding their condition rather than being 'decoupled' from such a discussion by the expert system of the doctor (Arntson and Droge, 1987). Once this oppositional force is in position, the issue for doctors then becomes one of how far they are prepared to take the subjectivity of the patient seriously, rather than seeing it as an impediment to their diagnostic and therapeutic understandings (Williams and Popay, 1994).

While the work of Giddens, Beck and Habermas emphasises the social factors which may be leading to a re-ordering of the doctor–patient relationship, other approaches focus more on the role of the market as the source of possible challenge. Over the past two decades, studies of health consumerism have introduced an economic scepticism into the debate around the supposed inevitability of asymmetry in the traditional relationship. In an American context, Haug and Levin approach the issue by asserting that a consumerist stance

> focuses on the purchaser's (patient's) rights and the seller's (physician's) obligations, rather than on the physician's rights (to direct) and the patient's obligations (to follow directions) … . In a consumer relationship, the seller has no particular authority; if anything, legitimated power rests in the buyer who can make the decision to buy or not to buy as he or she sees fit. (Haug and Levin, 1981: 213)

Behind this stance lies an assumption that 'consumerism implies the buyer's challenge of the seller's claims … an approach of doubt and caution, rather than faith and trust, in any transaction including the medical' (Haug and Levin, 1983: 10). While recognising that the absence of a price mechanism in the NHS diminishes the technical significance of this approach, nonetheless the consumerist values which are embodied in these statements have been much encouraged by successive governments from the introduction of the internal market in 1991 onwards. A health consumerist ideology has been propagated unconstrained by the market mechanism of responsibility to pay (see Chapter 3). Hence, patient expectations have taken on a consumerist quality with a consequent impact on the way in which patient demand registers in the doctor–patient relationship. A consumer frame of mind is particularly evident in the case of initial consultations, diagnostic tests and elective surgery where waiting lists are the norm.

With the fraying of the edges between public and private health care, patients are more prepared to move between them and, as a result, health consumerism is becoming a common feature of what were previously distinct sectors (see Chapter 6). As consumers become more accustomed to making health care choices, so they face issues common to their relationship with other types of service agencies and do not necessarily view asymmetries of knowledge as an insuperable difficulty. In this context, reflecting on the supposed vulnerability of private health care consumers, Wiles and Higgins note that they nonetheless exercise choice: 'While patients in this study had large gaps in their knowledge about costs, value for money, quality and options in private health care they did, nevertheless, express some preferences in the marketplace and secure services which they valued, at a time and place to suit their needs' (Wiles and Higgins, 1992: 80).

As one moves away from the medical stronghold of the NHS and conventional medicine towards complementary and alternative medicine (CAM), so the evidence increases of active health care consumers prepared to purchase the service they want rather than relying exclusively on the advice of doctors. In 1993, 33 per cent of the UK population were found to have used some form of complementary medicine and 10 per cent had consulted a complementary practitioner in the previous year. In addition, surveys of patients with chronic and difficult-to-manage diseases – such as cancer, HIV infection, multiple sclerosis, psoriasis and rheumatological conditions – identified levels of use which were twice as high (Zollman and Vickers, 1999a: 836). Furthermore, levels of use are increasing. Whilst in 1993 there were approximately 12 million adult consultations, in 1997 this had risen to an estimated 15 million consultations – 5 per cent of the number of general practice consultations. This picture of expanding activity is reinforced by the increase in the number of registered complementary practitioners in the UK from about 13 500 in 1991 to about 40 000 in 1997 (Zollman and Vickers, 1999a: 838; see also Sharma, 1995: 14–15).

International data supports the finding of a health care consumer prepared to move beyond the orbit of the traditional doctor–patient relationship. The proportion of the population who had used complementary therapies during the prior 12 months was estimated to be 10 per cent in Denmark in 1987 (Rasmussen and Morgall, 1990), 33 per cent in Finland in 1982 (Vaskilampi *et al.*, 1993), 49 per cent in Australia in 1993 (MacLennan *et al.*, 1996) and 15 per cent in Canada in 1995 (Millar, 1997). In the US, Eisenberg *et al.* found that between 1990 and 1997 the total visits to alternative medical practitioners (defined as a specific list of 16 therapies) had increased by 47 per cent from 427 million to 629 million, thereby exceeding total visits to all US primary care physicians. This is big business. Expenditure on alternative professional medical services rose by 47 per cent in the same period to an estimated \$21.2 billion with at least \$12.2 billion paid out of pocket – in other words as a direct cost to the consumer rather than indirect via an insurer. As the researchers observe, 'the magnitude of the demand for alternative therapies is noteworthy in light of the relatively low rates of insurance coverage for these services'. They continue, 'because the demand for health care (and presumably alternative therapies) is sensitive to how much patients must pay out of pocket, current use is likely to underrepresent utilisation patterns if insurance coverage for alternative therapies increases' (Eisenberg *et al.*, 1998: 1575).

The reasons given for the increased use of complementary medicine offer revealing insights into the changing nature of the relationship between patients and doctors. Research conducted in the 1980s presented people who use complementary therapies as 'mostly refugees from conventional medicine' (Fulder, 1988: 30), as passive actors who were pushed towards such therapies as a result of negative past experiences rather than pulled by their belief in the value of complementary care (Furnham and Smith, 1988). In contrast to this, later studies in the 1990s have found a medley of values at work as people decide to use complementary therapies as a matter of active choice rather than by default. Interestingly, it is the quality of the relationship with the complementary practitioner which receives most attention. Patients cite the amount of time available for the consultation and contrast this with the experience of seeing conventional NHS doctors, the attention given to the personality and experience of the patient, the increased opportunities for active patient participation in the process of recovery, and the resonance between the modes of explanation of a condition offered by a therapist and the beliefs and expectations of the patient (Zollman and Vickers, 1999b: 1488–9). In the experience of complementary therapy, there is felt to be less of a gap between the worlds of patient and practitioner than is the case in the conventional patient–doctor relationship (Vincent and Furnham, 1996). As a result, patients view the therapeutic encounter with complementary practitioners as more satisfying, empathetic and informative than that with their general practitioner (Ernst *et al.*, 1997). Furthermore, there is some evidence that they also see it as more effective in the treatment of specific conditions. A survey of musculoskeletal pain sufferers suggested that complementary treatments were perceived as more successful than mainstream drugs (Chrubasik *et al.*, 1998; quoted by Ernst, 1999: 1).

Whether the choice of complementary health care has an ideological as well as a pragmatic foundation, and therefore how coherent the opposition to conventional medicine may be, is not clear. Some have argued that the use of complementary therapies is associated with concepts of healing which emphasise the unity of body, mind and spirit, individual responsibility, anti-professionalism, self-care and personal transformation (Goldstein, 1992; Pauluch *et al.*, 1994). Whilst this may have some validity in some cases, more convincing is the argument that the increasingly pervasive values are those of what Kelner and Wellman term the 'smart consumers'. Rather than relying on institutional legitimacy as the basis for making their choice (i.e. the medical profession, hospitals, clinics) such consumers rely on their personal judgement and are prepared to move between conventional and complementary care as they see fit, choosing specific kinds of practitioners for particular problems (Kelner and Wellman, 1997: 211). In adopting this approach, consumers have in effect sought to redefine the doctor–patient relationship in terms of the patient as purchaser and the doctor as seller.

The industry of health care products is a willing ally of the emerging health care consumer and happy to help prise apart the patient–doctor relationship. Traditionally the sanctity of that relationship coupled with the interest of state and private insurance funding agencies to limit demand have acted as a barrier between industry and consumer. However, although in Europe the controls are as yet still in place, in the USA the Federal Drugs Agency (FDA) in 1985 lifted its moratorium on direct-to-consumer (DTC) advertising of prescription medicines and, with the arrival of the internet, pharmaceutical companies have been able to access consumers directly and with ease. In bypassing the information-gatekeeping role of the doctor, it is obviously in the industry's interest to encourage a situation where demand is driven by the consumer rather than the professional. And with consumers increasingly prepared to use the internet not only to access health information but also to inform their health care decisions, the obstacles to industry's ambition are not immediately apparent (Powell, 2002). As Sullivan observes of this phenomenon, 'the doctor–patient relationship of the future has many interested parties' and is becoming highly contested territory as these parties mount their different challenges to the dominance of conventional medicine (Sullivan, 2000: 401).

The continuities

In less than a generation, sociological theories and empirical evidence have combined to suggest that the traditional doctor–patient relationship is being radically, and successfully, challenged by a variety of social and economic developments. Asymmetric knowledge is now questionable if not obsolete, experts are losing their authority and patients are considered by many commentators to be 'expert', 'resourceful' and (like professionals) 'autonomous' in the health marketplace (see e.g. Coulter, 2002; Gray, 2002). While such impressive shifts make excellent academic copy, one should allow for the possibility that an embedded social institution such as medicine is capable of responding to challenge in ways that are adaptive and able to redefine the doctor–patient relationship so that the fundamentals of medical power are retained. Some compromises may be made, but not others. Political continuities may coexist with the processes of social change.

For the profession, it is important that, while concessions may be made, it retains its allegiance to scientific medical knowledge and the allopathic tradition. From this commitment derives its particular claim to authority and its distinctive approach to the doctor–patient relationship. The need for the protection of the knowledge base and the social power that flows from it has meant that the response to complementary and alternative medicine has been at best sceptical and at worst damning. Historically, the profession has diligently patrolled the boundaries of its NHS and private conventional medicine territories to ensure either that complementary medicine is debarred from entry or that it is allowed entry on condition that it does not threaten the traditional patient–doctor relationship. In other words, complementary medicine must accept the political rules governing the territory to which it has been granted admittance.

The principal justification for these immigration controls is a straightforward statement of professional ideology: that conventional medical practice is based on rigorously applied scientific knowledge and research, and complementary medicine is not. Beyond this, the more virulent attacks, particularly in the 1970s, emphasised that complementary medicine possesses none of the normal characteristics of a scientific culture in that it is irrational, lacks safety, encourages the transmission of disease, and is populist and sensationalist (Saks, 1995: 234–5). Supporting the ideological barriers were a range of practical measures designed to promote market exclusion. As one would expect, it was a central tenet of the historic concordat between medicine and the state that the latter would not provide legal or financial assistance to the former's competitors. Decades of lobbying for the state registration of different types of complementary medicine (as a means for acquiring social legitimacy) produced little effect in the face of the intransigent opposition of the medical establishment. It was not until the mid-1990s that two Acts of Parliament created the General Osteopathic Council and the General Chiropractic Council, an innovation which is the exception that proves the rule and is unlikely to be repeated. Other groups such as acupuncture and homeopathy have lobbied in vain for legislative sanction for their self-regulatory arrangements. It is worth noting also that although the osteopaths and chiropractors have achieved a measure of state recognition, this has not prevented the medical profession from vigorously rejecting their attempts to achieve a different form of respectability by becoming part of the professions allied to medicine (Saks, 1995: 195).

Within the NHS, any admittance of complementary medicine has been dependent on the grace and favour of the medical profession. Until relatively recently, doctors resisted the entry of any rivals into their NHS domain unless the complementary practitioners were able to demonstrate their scientific credentials. However to do so, practitioners need to have conducted research (for which support from the medically dominated funding agencies such as the Medical Research Council [MRC] was not forthcoming) and published in respectable medical journals (whose editors were reluctant to include the work of non-doctors) (Saks, 1995: 192–5). As a result, for many years the only way in which a complementary therapy could gain access to the NHS market was through active medical sponsorship which was given on a selective and highly conditional basis amounting, effectively, to colonisation. Thus in 1980, for example, the British Medical Acupuncture Society was set up to promote the use and scientific understanding of acupuncture as part of the practice of medicine. (It is a striking tribute to medical power that under the Medical Act of 1858 conventionally trained doctors can legally administer *any* unconventional medical treatments they choose provided what they do is acceptable to the legal principle of the 'Bolam test' which states that 'a doctor is not guilty of negligence if he or she has acted in accordance with a practice accepted as proper by a responsible body of medical men skilled in that particular art as long as it is subject to logical analysis' — as pure a statement of internalist governance values as one could wish to find (Zollman and Vickers, 1999c: 903). With an exclusively medical membership, which between 1980 and 1992 rose from 50 to 1000, its practitioners focused on the very restricted use of acupuncture as an alternative to surgical anaesthesia and as a means for alleviating painful conditions. Such an approach enabled them to use scientific methods to explain the effects of acupuncture in terms of medical theory and so retain their status as orthodox, and respected, doctors.

However, by the 1990s the rapid rise of CAM's market power was beginning to erode the profession's confidence in its imposition of rigid limitations on the presence of non-conventional medicines in the doctor–patient relationship. It was becoming clear that a more sophisticated response to this particular challenge was required. As a leading researcher into complementary medicine has observed, it is difficult for doctors to avoid the conclusion that 'CM's [complementary medicine's] popularity amounts to a biting criticism of mainstream medicine that ought to be taken seriously' (Ernst, 1999: 1). General practitioners have been particularly sensitive to the issue, perhaps because they are more exposed to direct, unfiltered consumer demands than are hospital doctors. As private business, they sit outside the main NHS bureaucracy and have continuous contact with a range of health consumers which may well encourage them to be more responsive to their views and preferences. Even in 1986, a survey of GPs in Oxfordshire found that 41 per cent believed that alternative systems of medicine were valid, 31 per cent claimed a working knowledge of at least one therapy and 50 per cent had delegated care of patients to lay practitioners (Anderson and Anderson, 1987; quoted by BMA, 1994: 35). Official NHS approval for this shift away from the traditional medical hostility to non-conventional medicine came in 1991 when GP Fundholders were given the power to award contracts for complementary therapy. In 1995, it was reported that over 20 per cent of primary health care teams provided some form of complementary medicine directly and, a year later, that 58 per cent of Primary Care Groups (PCGs) supplied access to complementary medicine (Laurent, 2000; Zollman and Vickers, 1999c: 901).

It is likely that the medical profession's move towards greater inclusiveness with regard to complementary medicine is based on market pragmatism rather than on any fundamental misgivings over the pre-eminence of medical science in the doctor–patient relationship. It is noticeable that it is the complementary therapies which have been legitimised by medical researchers that more commonly form part of the doctor's agenda. Osteopathy, acupuncture and some herbal medicines, for example, have become more acceptable to orthodox medicine as scientific research has begun to show how and why they achieve their therapeutic effect (Ernst, 2000; Saks, 1995: 239). Patients, however, value complementary medicines for different and often far more subjective reasons. Doctors are therefore left with the uneasy task of reconciling the difference between the belief system which informs their own decisions and the values on which their patients may draw in making their choices.

In the case of complementary medicine, and in areas of orthodox medicine where the patient is well informed, it can be argued that doctors need to develop an aspect to their role which recognises the rights of the patient as a consumer but retains the authority to enable the patient's choice to be made in a particular way. If they do not, then their political control of the relationship will be diminished. One option is that of the doctor as 'broker' or 'learned intermediary'. As Zollman and Vickers put it, 'A doctor who listens and supports patient choice, and whose advice minimises risk, rather than dismisses complementary medicine on principle, is more likely to encourage patients to use it appropriately, *as an adjunct*, rather than an alternative to conventional care' (Zollman and Vickers, 1999d: 1560, emphasis added). (Such a role is naturally based on the assumption that complementary medicine has a subordinate or secondary status to orthodox medicine.) Of course, in order to carry out this role and thus reconcile the 'two worlds' of orthodox and complementary medicine, doctors must acquire sufficient knowledge to 'guide their patients through the CM maze' (Ernst, 1999: 2). Once again the patient is dependent, but the dependency has been reformulated to incorporate a subdued version of patient choice.

A major limitation of this view of the adaptive doctor is the premium it places on the rationality of the doctor–patient interaction. In this sense there is, as Lupton points out, congruence between the notions of the 'consumerist' patient and the 'reflexive' actor and the understandings thus offered of possible change in the doctor–patient relationship. Both roles are understood as actively calculating, assessing and countering expert medical knowledge. Furthermore,

> neither approach tends to take into account the role played by cultural, psychodynamic and affective processes in individuals' everyday life choices, decisions and actions. That is, there is little understanding of the consumption of health care *qua* commodity as a dynamic and intersubjective sociocultural process rather than as an outcome of an individualised calculation. (Lupton, 1997: 374)

Thus in constructing understandings of how medical power works in the doctor–patient encounter, insufficient attention is paid to the emotional dependence of patients on doctors (often unarticulated), their desire for passivity rather than empowerment and their appreciation of routinised interactions. Behind this omission, typical most notably of the work of Giddens and Beck, lies the valuing of rational thought over the affective domain and the devaluing of emotionally based trust.

Once the doctor–patient relationship is seen less as an engagement between rational actors and more as an intersubjective interaction influenced by a variety of human needs and qualities, a less linear view of micro-medical power can be constructed where both traditional and challenging elements exist side by side. In his account of the changing doctor–patient relationship between 1930 and 1980, Armstrong notes that 'Whereas earlier the diagnostic function of medicine had created categories of patients with different diseases, the new medical gaze which created a web of observation and concern around the idiosyncratic patient established an individual identity' (Armstrong, 1982: 116). For medicine, patients now had an identity and that identity had to be included and negotiated within the medical organisation of the doctor–patient relationship. This shift was supported by a patient-centred medical discourse about the appropriate methods and skills to be used in the consultation in the course of which the subjective world of the patient was given credence, constituent qualities and status as the doctor accepted the patient-as-person (see e.g. Hopkins, 1972). In the case of general practice, the 'patient centred medicine' movement seeks, in the words of one of its standard texts, 'to empower the patient, to share power in the relationship; this means renouncing control that has been in the hands of the professional' (Stewart *et al.*, 1995: xvi).

Yet, it can be construed as change with an internal dynamic of political continuity. Commenting on this movement, Bloor contends that 'the GP is indeed renouncing control, but is also exchanging one kind of power relationship for another: the patient centred consultation is artfully contrived, bounded and orchestrated by the practitioner'. This, he maintains, parallels the situation in therapeutic communities where the characteristics of participative democracy are 'orchestrated by staff whose therapeutic gaze, like Foucault's, doesn't just see: it also governs, with patient participation being bounded, elicited, encouraged, overseen and rewarded' (Bloor, 2001: 33). As always in the doctor–patient relationship, the continuity in the medical project is the construction of public trust in medicine.

Conclusions

As Foucault points out, we continue to 'describe the effects of power in negative terms: it "excludes", it "represses", it "censors", it "abstracts", it "masks", it "conceals" '. In fact, he suggests, 'power produces; it produces reality; it produces domains of objects and rituals of truth. The individual and the knowledge that may be gained of him belong to this production' (Foucault, 1977: 194). With regard to the doctor–patient relationship, this is an important insight because it de-emphasises the simple dichotomies contained in the notions of asymmetric knowledge, paternalism versus patient empowerment, and so on. What this chapter has shown instead is that medical power in that relationship is complex, reflexive and mobile.

Its complexity derives from its ability to combine, and re-combine, rational and affective elements in endless patterns of interaction. Its focus may move from the objectivities of disease to the subjective world of the patient and back again. For doctors, unlike some sociologists, uncertainty is not a new idea but a continuity in the way in which medical knowledge is traded between themselves and patients. Ultimately, patients need a decision to be made about their condition to remove uncertainty and the role of the doctor is to make or enable that decision following an engagement with medical knowledge. The power of the doctor derives from the fact that without him no decision could be made, regardless of whether it is actually the patient or doctor who 'decides'. Thus, the truly autonomous patient would be one who was not a patient – that is, not dependent on the doctor for a decision to be made. The expert patient, on the other hand, would be one whose expertise formed part of the decision making process.

For medicine to retain its political control, both the social locale and the intersubjective relationship between the worlds of doctor and patient need to support the right of the doctor to determine what is, and what is not, a legitimate medical decision. The reflexivity of the doctor–patient relationship means that these social and intersubjective conditions can be fulfilled in many ways. The doctor may be paternalistic or enabling, the patient passive or proactive, or these characteristics may be combined in different ways within or between consultations. It matters not, so long as the patient 'trusts' the doctor.

In political terms, patient trust in doctors is a measure of the extent to which the process and outcome of the consultation is regarded as legitimate. The medical project is therefore continuously to find ways of constructing patient trust through the use of medical expertise and knowledge, emotional concern and empathy, and responsiveness to patient needs. In the course of the project, social patterns may be produced which can be characterised as 'the decline of paternalism', 'the rise of consumerism' or 'the challenge of the expert patient'. As yet, there is no evidence that any of these developments pose insoluble problems for medicine's reflexive capacity. Rather, they have demonstrated the political continuities of the profession's ability to engineer new rituals of truth in the nuanced context of the doctor–patient relationship.

3 The illusion of patient power

Introduction

At the sociological and cultural levels, it is clear that changes are taking place in the relationship between civil society and medicine. Health care consumers are making their choices in the health marketplace, patients are challenging the traditional form of the patient–doctor relationship, and a variety of groups have emerged to channel the consequent energies into political form. However, whether these developments are then reflected in parallel shifts in the macro politics of health is another matter. The systemic pact between medicine and the state is not designed to be flexible, but durable. It is rooted in a Health Service historically accustomed to the dominance of doctors and dependent in many ways on powerful institutions of medical self-governance.

Yet, according to the official discourse of UK health policy, patients occupy a central position in the politics of the NHS. Seemingly propelled by widely reported inquiries into medical malpractice and increasingly sophisticated health consumer groups, policy makers now give the patient pride of place in the policy documents they produce. Adjustments to accommodate the patient interest are apparently being made across a range of policy arenas. To take one major example, *The NHS plan* promises that patients will have a greater say in their treatment, more information, wider choice, and efficient means for redress, whilst professionals will be more responsive to patients' views and managers more diligently facilitating of the patient interest (Department of Health, 2000b: 88–95). With the NHS Reform and Health Care Professions Act 2002, the patient interest has been given statutory and bureaucratic reality in the form of Patient Forums and the Commission for

Patient and Public Involvement in Health. Patients, it would seem, have acquired a power base in the UK health policy community.

If true, this represents a significant shift in the balance of power between civil society, medicine and the state. But to what extent does the rhetoric of policy provide a sure guide to the politics of health? What measures should we use to gauge whether there has been a real change in medicine's traditional hegemony in this field? A key measure is the extent to which the policy community of health has adapted its established membership and procedures to incorporate the politically assertive health care consumer at the expense of the medical profession. If this has occurred, it will not be a new phenomenon. There are, for example, strong parallels between health policy today and food policy in the late 1980s where, under pressure from the outbreak of salmonella in eggs and other food scares, the consensual policy community was obliged to evolve into more pluralistic 'issue networks' to deal with consumer pressures (Smith, 1991). If this transformation is beginning to occur in the health policy arena, then we would expect it to be signalled by a growth in patient-based policy networks, a shift in the dominant ideology of the policy community (and in particular the values of the medical profession) towards an acceptance of an enhanced role for patients in policy making, a growing interaction between patient policy networks and policy decision makers, and, most importantly, patient influence over the allocation of resources.

This chapter begins by examining the relationship between patients and the orthodox policy community of the NHS dominated by the medical profession, the politicians, the policy makers and, to a lesser extent, the managers. In particular, it is impossible to conceive of a sustainable change in the power of patients without a corresponding shift in the power of doctors. Doctors dispose of NHS resources to patients on the basis of a medical authority rooted in ideological and structural assumptions ingrained in the operation of the NHS and its policy community. If the subordinate power position of patients is to be transformed, these assumptions will have to be challenged. Second, therefore, to what extent does such a challenge exist, what are its ideological roots, and how far does it engage with the central issue of medical power in the health policy community? Assuming that the challenge is manifest in the form of new health consumer policy networks, a third issue then arises. What has been the policy community's response to patient demands for inclusion – have they become equal partners in the politics of that community, or have they simply been accommodated in ways which preserve the traditional distribution of medical power?

A stable policy community

Stable policy communities emerge when the state's engagement with a particular set of policy networks becomes routinised, boundaries are established to identify 'insiders' and 'outsiders' in the policy domain, and a policy paradigm is institutionalised (e.g. Marsh and Smith, 2000; Wright, 1988). Underpinning the policy community are shared values, a common understanding of 'the rules of the game', trust between its members, and an acceptance that cooperation is the best way to achieve common goals (Borzel, 1998; Hindmoor, 1998). Once stability is established, a policy community may come to dominate all phases of the policy process: agenda setting, evaluation of alternatives, policy formulation, policy implementation and policy evaluation (Coleman, 1999). To maintain that stability and the efficient delivery of policy, networks which do not share the values of the policy community are excluded or allowed only restricted and conditional access to the policy-making process.

Up to the late 1980s, UK health care was characterised by a closed policy community that exercised a firm control over policy agenda setting, formation and implementation. The policy networks of health consumer groups were non-existent, passive or medically dominated (e.g. disease-based associations). What Haywood and Hunter described as 'the iron triangle' of the medical profession, ministers and officials ensured that although differences might arise they could be resolved through the use of formal and informal networks (Haywood and Hunter, 1982; see also Ham 1985: 97–9). Policy was framed within a set of values that constituted a form of 'ideological corporatism' so completely dominated by the medical profession that it has been described by some as an example of 'the professionalised state' where the state effectively delegates power and responsibility for a policy area to a particular professional group (Dunleavy, 1981: 8–9; Dunleavy and O'Leary, 1987: 320–3). For the principal parties concerned, it was an arrangement based on an exchange of macro-political benefits. On the one hand, the state was able to rely on the medical profession both to provide citizens with their health care rights and to manage the tensions between the demand for health care and the available supply. On the other, by fulfilling its obligations to both state and citizens and maintaining an appropriate standard of care, the medical profession continued to justify its right, granted by the state, to the privilege of self-regulation and its associated social and economic advantages (see Chapter 1).

What may be termed the political culture of the NHS necessarily supported the policy community of medicine and state through an assumptive world of beliefs and actions. As a consequence, even when the historic agreement between medicine and state became unstable, the ability of government to implement policies at variance with the tenets of that agreement was limited by the inertia of the NHS's traditional political culture. It is a political culture founded on the assumed pre-eminence of medical authority in the doctor–patient relationship. That authority is derived from the profession's control of a body of scientific knowledge which is seen by the public as high status, socially functional and, above all, legitimate. As a result the public 'trusts' the profession, which, in political terms, can be taken to mean that the public gives doctors the power to exercise a wide discretion in the diagnosis of the condition, the definition of the therapeutic treatment and, in consequence, the allocation of the health care resources required for that treatment. Individual control of the body is relinquished and becomes part of the medical domain, owned and disposed of by doctors. Regardless of the organisational context, this essential power relationship has the capacity to drive, or inhibit, the direction of change because it is the crucible within which is forged the supply–demand relationship in health care and from which flows the bargaining power of medicine with the state. Thus whilst the process of policy *formation* may adjust to pressures for greater patient power, how far those policies can be *implemented* will depend on the malleability of the patient–doctor relationship.

With the foundation of the NHS this culture was incorporated into an organisation where 'implicit in the structure' was a bargain between the state and the medical profession which guaranteed that 'while central government controlled the budget, doctors controlled what happened within that budget' (Klein, 1989: 82;

see also Salter, 1995); the policy community worked within a medically defined agenda on condition that doctors enabled the process of policy implementation. Patients were the presumed beneficiaries of the bargain, not participants in it. Economically secure for the first time in its history, the profession could rely on the NHS to construct a bureaucratic web which supported a medical definition of the mode and style of intercourse between patients and doctors. Meanwhile, the many and diverse institutions of medical self-regulation remained undisturbed, a tangible tribute to the power of doctors to retain control of their traditional territory whilst colonising another (see Chapter 5). Where specific NHS procedures were introduced for the regulation of doctors these were medically dominated, rarely invoked, and in no sense a vehicle for patient grievances (Allsop and Mulcahy, 1996: 37–72; Donaldson, 1994a). This was to be expected. Since the NHS bureaucracy happily embraced the principle that clinical autonomy acted in the interests of patients, there was no justification for inventing procedures which questioned both the principle and the medical decisions that flowed from it.

Destabilising the policy community

Given the longevity, strength and functionality of the UK policy community, new policy networks could not expect to be warmly embraced. If the stability of that community was to be seriously challenged, its values would need to be undermined, its legitimacy thus questioned, its networks penetrated and its political efficacy fragmented. Such a process would be lengthy, arduous and with no guarantee of success. Furthermore, the policy community could respond to the challenge in a variety of ways. It might seek to reject the challenge, fragment it, co-opt it on terms which suited the policy community's existing power arrangements, make cosmetic and symbolic adjustments, or, finally, reorganise the policy community's internal balance of power in order to incorporate the new interest. Much would depend on the internal relationships in the community and the degree of common purpose or tensions between its constituent partners.

Ideological pressure on the established policy community began with the rise of the New Right in British politics and its direct challenge to the NHS's traditional view of medical dominance in the doctor–patient relationship. In the mid-1980s, New Right intellectuals of the Conservative Party argued that market principles were as equally well suited to the provision of health care as they were to other areas of social policy (Elwell, 1986; Green, 1986, 1988; Letwin and Redwood, 1988). Their critique of the NHS suggested that bureaucratic inertia and professional dominance had produced a service unresponsive to the needs of the health care consumer. To correct this, they maintained, what was required was a devolution of money and power to the consumer, greater patient choice of health care provider, and a corresponding diminution of the power of both doctors and managers as competition becomes a reality. However, so long as the NHS remained the sacred and inviolable institution of the welfare state (the 'jewel in the crown'), the translation of the New Right's market principles into policy could not escape engagement with a profession and a bureaucracy to whom direct patient power was an alien concept. What was less alien was the creation of a new form of agency relationship between the patient, on the one hand, and the NHS bureaucracy and the medical profession, on the other. Thus *Working for patients*, the 1989 White Paper which launched the 'internal market' as it was known, established purchasing agencies to identify patient needs and commission the health care services to meet those needs through contracts with providers (Department of Health, 1989a).

However, by separating the customer role of payee (DHA, FHSA and GP Fundholder) from the consumer role of service recipient (patient), the new agency relationships simply created a novel form of patient dependency organised at the level of populations rather than individual patients and doctors. Patients were not given an organisational base or policy networks in the NHS, remained outside the NHS power structures and policy community, but new ways were invented to look after their interests.

Although the consumerist ambitions of the New Right were duly subordinated to professional and bureaucratic interest, they resonated strongly with an emergent ideological theme concerning the need for the NHS to be more open and accountable to citizens. Part of a broader critique of the 'democratic deficit' in government and the rise of 'the new magistracy' in public service management, this theme emphasises the inadequacies of representative democracy, the importance of continuing citizen participation in the accountability structures of the welfare state, and links between participation and institutional legitimacy (Hughes *et al.*, 1997; Stewart and Stoker, 1995). Thus, for example, the Association of Community Health Councils for England and Wales argues that 'the principal route in a democracy to close this kind of trust gap between the public and the institution [the NHS] is to promote its accountability and thereby secure its legitimacy'. It continues, 'the more accountable the NHS, the more the public's sense of its ownership and the more it is legitimate' (Association of Community Health Councils for England and Wales, 1999: 4).

Although rooted in the quite different value positions of the market and democracy, the themes of consumerism and citizen involvement both act to promote the significance of the patient as a player in the politics of the NHS and, *ipso facto*, constitute an ideological force against the traditional dominance of doctors in the policy community. However, the translation of general ideological shifts into a power advantage for particular groups is dependent in the first instance on policy networks capable of exploiting the new values in the context of particular issues and what Kingdon calls 'the policy window', where an opportunity occurs allowing problem, policy and political streams to be brought together (Kingdon, 1984).

As a possible platform for oppositional behaviour, user and carer self-help groups can provide their members with 'the opportunities, stories and sets of behaviour to increase their perceived control over their physical and social conditions' (Arntson and Droge, 1987; quoted by Kelleher, 1994: 109). In so doing, they create a life-world where there is the opportunity to discuss the experience of chronic illness through a discourse which uses a moral and practical form of reasoning as opposed to the language of expert systems (Kelleher, 1994: 114–15). By creating a social identity based on their own definition of their condition, or the condition of those for whom they care, such groups have enabled their members to challenge the medically dominated institutional and service assumptions which circumscribe the delivery of care (Sang, 2000). However, whether at the political level their challenge to the values and organisation of conventional NHS medicine has then been translated into policy networks with access to the policy community is debatable. Wood's research on orthodox, disease-based patients' associations found that, at the local level, they usually lack political legitimacy in the eyes of Health Authorities, which prefer to rely instead on consultative methods (Wood, 2000: 14). Exceptions to this rule, he argues, are the overtly political activities of the feminist, disability and AIDs lobbies which, unlike the more traditional patients' associations, adopt a vigorous campaigning style in order to achieve maximum visibility and impact.

An alternative view is that high profile political activity, rather than being the exception, is in fact the characteristic of an emergent sector of health consumer politics characterised by new and dynamic policy networks. At present there are about 2500 user and carer groups listed on the database of the College of Health, and their numbers and complexity are growing as consumers discover new ways of organising and expressing their interests (Sang, 2000: 22). The traditional patients' associations with their frequent ties to medical specialties have been outstripped (in numbers at least) by service user groups (e.g. Survivors Speak Out, Mindlink), condition-related groups (e.g. National Schizophrenic Fellowship, Manic Depression Fellowship, Depression Alliance) and advocacy groups (e.g. UK Advocacy Network). However, the existence of large numbers of vocal health consumer groups does not, of itself, mean that the policy community will feel obliged to listen to them. A policy window is required.

In the UK that window of opportunity has taken the form of the politicisation of medical regulation following the high-profile case of the three Bristol consultants disciplined by the GMC for professional misconduct and the associated public inquiry (Bristol Royal Infirmary Inquiry, 2000), the inquiry into organ retention at Alder Hey Children's Hospital Liverpool (Royal Liverpool Children's Hospital Inquiry, 2001), the case of the GP Harold Shipman who received 15 life sentences for murdering 15 of his middle-aged and elderly women patients by lethal injections of diamorphine, and the regular reports of incompetent doctors (see Chapter 6). As in other policy fields, the media has been the key instrument in taking the low-profile issue of the regulation of doctors, giving it visibility, putting and keeping it on the agenda of the policy community, facilitating the development of health consumer policy networks, and monitoring the policy community's response (McCombs and Shaw, 1972; Protess and McCombs, 1991). Issue-based groups such as Bristol Heart Children's Action Group (BCAG), Parents Interring Their Young Twice (PITY II – Alder

Hey), and the National Committee Relating to Organ Retention (NCAOR) have assiduously used media interest in an attempt to gain access to the policy community and help shape the spirit, if not the details, of the policy agenda on medical regulation.

A window of opportunity had clearly arrived. However, who would exploit it and how would they do it? Could it act as a vehicle for the reformulation of the policy community and the inclusion of patient power? To answer this question we need first to consider how and why the policy community has responded to the general pressures for greater patient involvement over the past 15 years, what effect this has had on the internal balance of power within the community, and therefore how it might respond to the latest set of political demands from health consumers.

Reformulating the policy community

In the late 1980s, the promotion by the state of managers as a power group to rival doctors was followed by the exclusion of the medical profession from the inner sanctum of policy making during the intense activities which accompanied the formulation of the internal market policy (Butler, 1992; Lee-Potter, 1997). Armed with the anti-profession ideology of the New Right, the Conservative government sought to rebalance the policy community in the favour of managers and politicians. Yet, it did so largely in terms of policy *formation*. The ability of doctors to hinder or facilitate policy *implementation* remained unchecked. Medicine's entire system of autonomous professional governance continued on its serene, unaccountable course, a separate and parallel system of power within the NHS with which all service delivery policies must engage in one way or another. Even the drive to reduce medicine's influence over policy formation soon lost its impetus. By the mid-1990s there were strong indications that the state had learnt the error of its ways, realised the fundamental importance of a high-level political bargain with medicine, publicly transformed managers from heroes into villains, and was returning to a grudging acceptance of the importance of the medical profession to the efficient operation of the policy community (Hunter, 1994; Klein, 1995).

Despite the Conservative government's rhetoric regarding the importance of patients, this had never been construed by politicians as meaning that health consumers should therefore form part of the health policy community. In the early and mid-1990s, the recognition that strategies for the political inclusion of patients in NHS policy making were desirable as a means for conferring legitimacy on policy outcomes was tempered by a wariness among managers, doctors and politicians about the possible destabilising effects of such strategies on the policy community. It was fairly predictable, therefore, that the approach adopted was consultative, strong on rhetoric, and ambiguous in its commitment to patient influence. Thus the guidance on public involvement in the purchasing function issued as part of the internal market reforms stated that: 'Being responsive to local views will enhance the credibility of health authorities but, more importantly, is likely to result in services which are better suited to local needs and therefore more appropriate.' But continued: 'There may of course be occasions when local views have to be over-ridden (e.g. the weight of epidemiological, resource or other considerations) and in such circumstances it is important that health authorities explain the reasons for their decisions' (National Health Service Executive, 1992: 3). In practice, purchasing agencies differed widely in the extent to which they promoted local involvement (if at all), the methods used (e.g. surveys, health panels, focus groups, citizen juries), the issues addressed, and the significance attached to the data gathered (Donaldson, 1995; Milewa *et al.*, 1998). What Harrison and Mort have described in their research as 'a consultation industry' developed, with no firm commitment given to abide by the results of the consultation, and with local NHS managers treating user groups 'as a recognised feature of the organisational landscape, but not one to which any superior degree of legitimacy was accorded' (Harrison and Mort, 1998: 66). For the most part the experiments with patient involvement were confined to the local level. They can perhaps be best described as a form of 'sponsored consumerism' where there is a controlled inclusion of patients in the policy process – but on the periphery of the policy community and in the context of an already agreed policy agenda.

Although the direct ideological challenge of radical Conservatism to the dominant doctor and the passive patient had evaporated, that of New Labour was soon to arrive. Equally suspicious of the privileged professional, equally attentive to the needs of the consumer, the Labour government appeared ready to re-engineer the dominant forces in the policy community for both policy formation *and* implementation. Add to this the political impetus generated by the events at Bristol, Alder Hey and elsewhere, and the window of opportunity offered by the politicisation of medical regulation, and once again it seemed as if medicine was about to be marginalised. Surely, it seemed, the era of 'sponsored consumerism' was now anachronistic and about to be replaced by an explicit incorporation of the patient interest into the policy community.

Guided both by the political need to respond to these events, and by a keen sense of an opportunity to outflank the medical profession, politicians and their policy makers have made 'patient empowerment' a central ideological symbol of all their major health policies since 1998. As in other policy spheres, the objective is to legitimise policy making by the use of a political language which constantly reiterates a particular theme: in this case, that the public plays a central role in both the policy process and its outcomes. To the extent that the symbols embedded in that language are accepted as part of the dominant political discourse, their legitimising effect is strengthened, that is, the political advantage they offer is increased (Edelman, 1985, 1988).

For example, *The NHS plan* (a ten-year strategy) begins with its vision of a health service 'designed around the patient', and in a subsequent chapter details how patients will have new rights and roles, more say in their treatment, and more influence over the way the NHS works. They are to be empowered through more information, more choice, better protection, more rights of redress, a new patient advocacy and liaison service, and the creation in each health authority of patient forums with the ability to elect representatives to local trust boards (Department of Health, 2000b: 88–95). Similarly, the recommendations of the Bristol Royal Infirmary Inquiry's final report are based on the premise that 'the patient must be at the heart of everything the NHS does', as are the objectives of the latest (2002) reorganisation of the NHS where it is reiterated that patients must influence both the shape and the delivery of their health care (Bristol Royal Infirmary Inquiry, 2000: 435; Department of Health, 2002i: 3). Even clinical diagnosis and treatment, the very heart of medical power, are presented (at least in policy terms) as arenas where health professionals are encouraged 'to treat patients as equal partners in the decision making process' (Department of Health, 2000e: i). Such is the symbolic potency of the elixir of patient empowerment that it is claimed it will enhance service quality, strengthen public confidence in the NHS and, by some mysterious process, improve individual and population health (Department of Health, 2000e: 3). In the case of research, where a Standing Group on Consumers in NHS Research has existed since 1996, it is believed that consumer involvement in all stages of research will lead to research which is more relevant to the needs of consumers, more reliable, and more likely to be used (National Health Service Executive, 1999e: 6).

The state's intense ideological promotion of the patient interest has been matched by its production of a range of policies designed to restrict the traditional autonomy of doctors (see Chapter 6). In the consultation document *A first class service: quality in the new NHS*, the government proposed a comprehensive, management-led system of clinical governance designed to set and monitor clinical standards (Department of Health, 1998b). Even the traditional independence of GPs is to be limited by the ambition of Primary Care Trusts (PCTs) to bring clinical governance within the managerial orbit. Self-regulation remains, but the document notes that if public confidence in doctors is to be restored, self-regulation must be modernised to ensure that it is 'open to public scrutiny; responsive to changing clinical practice and changing service needs; and publicly accountable for professional standards set nationally and the action taken to maintain those standards' (Department of Health, 1998b: para 3.44). In effect, notice was given that medicine's system of governance was to be integrated with the normal procedures of NHS management, the profession's independence restricted, and its ability to inhibit policy implementation much reduced. Other measures have pursued the same agenda: clinical standards are to be set by the National Institute for Clinical Excellence (NICE) and the National Service Frameworks (NSFs); monitored by the Commission for Health Improvement (CHI), the NHS Performance Assessment Framework and the National Patient Survey; locally delivered through clinical governance systems; and 'underpinned' by the National Clinical Assessment Authority (NCAA) to deal with poorly performing doctors and the National Patient Safety Agency (NPSA) to facilitate learning from adverse events (Department of Health, 1999a, 2001a,i).

What does this avalanche of 'patient-friendly' statements and 'doctor-hostile' policies mean for the fundamental balance of power in the policy community? Despite the impressive weight of the bureaucratic inventions for the control of the medical profession, they still have to be made to work – which, as always, requires the cooperation of doctors, no matter how sophisticated the management arrangements. Ultimately, both consultants and GPs have the option of market exit from the NHS into the private sector, a move which might well increase rather than diminish their bargaining power. The logical difficulty therefore faced by the state is this: why should the medical profession help implement policies on the governance of medicine which would negate the profession's cardinal power position in the implementation of policy in general by restricting doctors' freedom of decision making? Given the importance attached by the government to the implementation of one very ambitious policy, the NHS Plan, this is clearly a sensitive question. The likely answer is that the profession may accept a repackaging and redefinition of its power, but only if it remains a dominant partner in the health policy community.

Independently of the health policy community, different parts of the medical profession have reacted in different ways to the pressures from health consumers for a reshaping of the patient–doctor relationship. Consultants, embedded as they are in the institutional heart of the NHS and surrounded by the technology of the scientific paradigm, have found it difficult to comprehend the cultural imperatives which drive their patients. For example, the outrage of parents whose children's body organs had been retained by consultants at Bristol Royal Infirmary and Alder Hey Hospital, Liverpool without their proper informed consent immediately encountered arguments from consultants about the importance of medical research and the need to maintain the flow of organs for that research. Lay and medical cultures confronted each other in a previously quiescent area of the doctor–patient relationship where medical authority had always been taken for granted so that the nature of consent had not been an issue (Bristol Royal Infirmary Inquiry, 2000; Royal Liverpool Children's Inquiry, 2001). Since the retention of body parts without the fully informed consent of relatives was soon shown by the Chief Medical Officer's subsequent inquiry to be common practice in many NHS hospitals as opposed to an exceptional incident, the issue served to illustrate dramatically the assumptive nature of the cultural divisions (Chief Medical Officer, 2001). As the Chief Medical Officer's report observed, with a commendable degree of understatement, 'it is the extent to which this [system for the retention of tissues and organs] has fallen out of step with public understanding and public expectations which is at the heart of the present controversy' (Chief Medical Officer, 2001: para 3.3). Both sides considered that they had the right to the use of the dead body. Such was intensity of the conflict that, after some prevarication and attempts at neutrality, the Secretary of State for Health was obliged to establish the official position on an unprecedented issue. Revealingly, in a statement accompanying the publication of the Alder Hey report, he came down firmly in favour of the lay view: 'We can no longer accept the traditional patronising attitude of the NHS that the benefits of medicine, science or research are somehow self-evident regardless of the wishes of patients or their families. There is a simple principle at stake here. The health of the patient belongs to the patient, not the health service' (Bale, 2001). Whether the majority of consultants would agree with such a bold refashioning of their traditional relationship with their patients is debatable.

Although the elites of medicine are undoubtedly aware that change is necessary, some are more aware than others. Not all would agree with the unequivocal statement from the Royal College of Anaesthetists that 'The culture of paternalism and deference has gone. People know more about health matters. They want to be well informed and involved in decisions about their medical care. They see themselves as partners with doctors in that process.' (Royal College of Anaesthetists and the Association of Anaesthetists of Great Britain and Ireland, 1998: 3.) In addition, the exclusion of patients from medicine's own policy community (apart from a variety of innocuous 'patient liaison' arrangements) mirrors the situation in the health policy community as a whole and inevitably restricts the agenda-setting options. As a consequence, medicine's recent policy discourse has almost invariably focused on how the assumptions of medical authority and autonomy can be retained in any reformed system of regulation rather than on an enhanced role for patients within it (see Chapter 6).

One possible exception to this general observation are general practitioners. On the reform of medical regulation, the Royal College of General Practitioners (RCGP) took the unusual line that 'if revalidation [of doctors] is to command the respect and support of the public, patients themselves must be actively involved in all stages of revalidation' (Royal College of General Practitioners, 1999: 6). This more open stance may reflect the fact that, in general, GPs are more exposed to direct, unfiltered consumer demands than are hospital doctors. As private businesses they sit outside the main NHS structures, have less bureaucratic protection than do consultants, and are therefore more responsive to consumer views and preferences.

The state's position would be less confined if it had alternative partners which it could draw into the policy community to offset the continuities of medical power. The limits of managerial power in implementing policies have been all too obviously exposed, not least by government ministers seeking scapegoats, and managers lack political and media credibility; but not so patients. So what is the likelihood that the state will move beyond the use of patient empowerment as a symbolic device, to recognise the validity of an independent patient voice and integrate the policy networks of health policy consumers into the routinised operation of the policy community?

The initial evidence is not promising. At the same time as *The NHS plan* enlarged the bureaucracy of sponsored consumerism, it also proposed the abolition of the Community Health Councils (CHCs), since 1974 the only independent source of consumer views in the NHS and a frequent irritant to local NHS managers (Adams, 1998). As such, the CHCs were never integrated into the policy community and, in the view of the Association of CHCs for England and Wales (ACHCEW), were deliberately shut out of the consultation process for *The NHS plan* (Greenwood, 2000). Other data indicate that this may simply mean that the CHCs are being superseded by more relevant health consumer networks. Health consumer groups were involved in the six modernisation teams which contributed to the drawing up of *The NHS plan*, and are represented on the taskforces which oversee its implementation and on the working groups of the NSFs which define the government's health priorities. Lay members are present on the new regulatory bodies such as CHI and NICE (Allsop *et al.*, 2002). Perhaps most significantly, the establishment by the NHS Reform and Health Care Professions Act 2002 of the Commission for Patient and Public Involvement in Health (CPPIH) and its associated local Patient Forums has created a statutory and bureaucratic vehicle for possible health consumer influence in the policy community. Accountable to the Secretary of State for Health and the Health Committee of the House of Commons, the CPPIH will have the independence of a Non-Departmental Public Body (NDPB) and the function of promoting health consumer involvement in the policy process (Transition Advisory Board, 2002).

It will be interesting to see how far the new arrangements are able to bring coherence to what research has shown to be the fragmented character of health consumer policy networks. Divided by objectives, interests, size, structure, strategy, tactics and degree of stability, health consumer groups have only recently begun to aggregate themselves into networks with resources (such as expertise) which policy makers need and value (Allsop *et al.*, 2002: 61). Umbrella organisations – such as the Long-term Medical Conditions Alliance and the Patients Forum (1988) – with the capacity to act as coordinators of the patient interest through their role as what Sabatier has termed 'advocacy coalitions', are few (Sabatier, 1988). On the other hand, policy makers may have begun to heed the logic of their own policy rhetoric. In one study, almost a third of the consumer groups surveyed believed that opportunities for participation in the health policy process had grown over the past three years (Jones *et al.*, 2000). However, by itself, consumer involvement in the policy process is no guarantee that the state has recognised the political utility of this contribution in anything other than a symbolic sense. It may be a form of co-option, not simply because the state wants to co-opt (which it may), but also because it will take time for the health consumer networks to develop their own particular niche in the workings of an established policy community, not to mention the political skills to match those of the medical profession, and thus provide a possible counterweight to medical power (Barnes, 1999; Saward, 1990).

The acid test of how far the state is prepared to redefine the relationship between itself, civil society and medicine by advancing the cause of health consumers as active participants in the policy process, is in the policy arena where the collision between patient and doctor interest has been most visible and most intense: medical regulation. It is notable that, despite the plethora of policy initiatives in this field, the mode of policy formation and implementation reflects the traditional policy community approach (see Chapter 6). Politicians and policy makers bargain with the elites of medicine to produce regulatory policies, managers attempt to implement them, and patients are assumed to be the grateful recipients of the policy outputs. For example, *Supporting doctors, protecting patients*, a key consultation document dealing with the operational details of the future system of medical regulation, barely mentions the contribution of patients, as it struggles to reconcile the state's management ambitions with the labyrinth of self-regulation (Department of Health, 1999a). Likewise, the reforms being introduced by the profession's self-regulatory bodies generally aim to improve their internal efficiency rather than open themselves to the external scrutiny of health consumers (Salter, 2001: 875–91). An exception to this is the GMC which registers UK doctors. Much of the political pressure generated by the politicisation of medical regulation has focused on the decisions and structure of the GMC, a key member of the health policy community. As a result, not only are patients being given an important role in its revised poor performance procedures and its proposed system of revalidation, but the proportion of lay members on its reformed Council has increased from 25 to 40 per cent (Department of Health, 2002d).

Conclusions

The pressure from health consumer groups of civil society for a greater role in policy making is not unique to the UK. In Canada a sustained patients' campaign in the 1980s produced a radically reformed system of medical regulation with increased layperson representation on the governing councils of medical colleges, and in the USA consumer, patient and advocate groups are now an established feature of the health care landscape (Coburn, 1993; Ross, 1999). Meanwhile in Europe, consumer groups are campaigning for comprehensive legislation on patients' rights in Denmark and Finland, as well as at the European Union level (Hogg, 1999: 140, 179). But what the UK experience tells us is that the translation of consumer pressure into significant power shifts in the health policy community is a complex process. Visibility in the political arena is no guarantee of civil society influence over the policies produced or the resources allocated.

In the UK, market and democratic ideological themes have lent support and credence to the emergence of health consumer groups.

At the same time, new issue networks have developed, stimulated by the policy window of opportunity associated with unprecedented media interest in the Bristol, Alder Hey and Harold Shipman cases, the continuing flow of 'dangerous doctor' stories, and the politicisation of medical regulation. The response of the health policy community to these pressures has been ambiguous. On the one hand, the mantra of patient empowerment now permeates the policy discourse, and patients have been given a statutory and bureaucratic presence in the NHS structure. On the other, the content of the reforms of medical regulation reflect the balance of forces within the existing health policy community from which patients were, and are, excluded. As a result of the introduction of new policies on clinical governance, doctors find themselves more accountable for their actions. However, that accountability is largely to other doctors and (notionally) to managers, not to patients.

Despite their differences, medicine and the state remain the dominant partners of the policy community and disinclined to destabilise it by incorporating the new and unpredictable policy networks of civil society. Thus, although the various regulatory policies produced may at times have the flavour of confrontation between the ambitions of state management and the recalcitrance of professional autonomy, both partners know that it is in their mutual interest to construct a consensus. The state needs the profession to implement policies which deal with the demands of its citizens, and the profession needs the state to continue to support its self-regulatory and market privileges. Whilst the health consumer policy networks remain fragmented and immature, and while the many variations of sponsored consumerism continue to legitimate policies, there is no incentive for the state to change its ways and incorporate the former into the agenda setting stage of policy formation. In any case, whilst the state has an interest in making the profession more accountable to the NHS managers (its allies), it has no interest in confusing the lines of accountability (and the negotiations) by insisting that doctors also be more accountable to their patients.

Medicine could choose to act independently of the state and itself recognise the emerging reality of the patient as health care consumer, rather than rely on government policymaking as the engine of change. The difficulty faced by such an initiative is that the governance of the profession is characterised by diverse institutions, frequently divided among themselves, which recognise no single locus of coordinating power (see Chapter 5). The elites of the GMC, Medical Royal Colleges, specialist associations, BMA and medical schools have enough difficulty determining their respective intra-professional contributions to any reformed system and then negotiating with the state without the additional complication of integrating new and inexperienced players into the bargaining process. So, although one part of the profession may be prepared to adapt to the political implications of a changed patient–doctor relationship, others will happily ignore them. Cultural change may be one thing, political change is quite another.

4 Doctors and managers

Introduction

In 1983, *The NHS management inquiry* chaired by Sir Roy Griffiths launched managers on their difficult voyage as a power group in the Health Service (Department of Health and Social Security, 1983a). In so doing, the inquiry issued a challenge to the established principle of medical hegemony which, in various policy guises, has regularly resurfaced in the following two decades. As the agents of the state in its attempts to refashion its historic concordat with the medical profession, managers have assumed the onerous burden of attempting to implement policies which seek to remove, limit or redefine the many and varied facets of entrenched medical power in the NHS. In response, the profession has ignored, blocked or reinterpreted policies as necessary to protect its power base.

The result is a continuing political struggle which, although it may take place within different health policy domains, has a number of key dimensions that provide a guide to the changing balance of power. In the course of that struggle, managers have found themselves cast at one time as the harbingers of rational progress and, at another, as the villains of the piece, the 'grey suits' who frustrate the good intentions of the men and women in 'white coats'. The politicians in particular have been inconstant allies, caught between their desire to downsize the power of medicine and their need for doctors to continue to deliver their political promises to citizens.

This chapter focuses on the engagement between doctors and managers in the years of the Conservative governments up to 1997 with Chapter 6 then taking up the story and tracing the rather different character of that relationship with Labour in power. It begins by analysing the historic construction of the management myth in the face of the continuing reality of medical power and its first manifestation in the form of general management in the 1980s. Second, it examines the re-launching of the management project as a key component of the 1990 internal market reforms and the intricacies of management's relationship with medicine in the secondary care sector. Faced with a vast agenda of change, how did managers deal with the political ambiguities inherent in their relative powerlessness when compared to the entrenched advantages of the medical profession? Third, what of primary care where NHS management was noticeable largely by its absence? What compromises were forced on a state faced with the independence of the general practitioner and how did the GP Fundholder policy impact on the management agenda?

Management as myth

The arrival of general management with the Griffiths Report in 1983 went totally against the grain of the traditional NHS culture. When founded in 1948, the NHS was the product of a high level political agreement between medicine and the state: the state gained a health care system to protect and regulate its populace and the medical profession gained money, status and the power to protect and regulate its privileges. That concordat was recognised at every level of the Health Service in terms of its values, structures and procedures and in terms of the NHS's engagement, or non-engagement, with the profession's system of self-regulation. Underpinning it were assumptions regarding the profession's clinical autonomy (the ability to dispose of clinical resources), economic autonomy (the ability to determine one's own system of economic rewards including market entry and exit) and political autonomy (the ability to determine important elements of health policy and its implementation) (see Chapter 1).

The exercise of these autonomies meant that large areas of NHS activity were under the control of a power group which was not accountable to NHS authority but to its own internal system of self-regulation. An appreciation of the broad sweep of territories involved is provided by Table 1.1. Starting from the defining characteristic of professional autonomy as control over a particular body of knowledge in terms of its creation (research), transmission (education) and application (performance), we can see that in the case of the Health Service the incorporation of these functional autonomies placed medicine in what, for decades, was an impregnable position. As a professional body, doctors were assumed to have the right to set their own standards, monitor their own behaviour, and implement their own corrective sanctions where necessary (see Chapter 5).

Within the ideology which supported this arrangement, doctors were seen to be acting purely in the interests of their patients, uninfluenced by non-clinical factors such as the resources available. Direct management of their activities by non-clinicians was unacceptable because it would undermine this understanding and, *ipso facto*, the basis of medical authority and public trust. If public trust was undermined, then so also would be the ability of the profession to deliver its part of the bargain with the state: the rationing of health care resources to civil society. Given the dominance of the medical hegemony and its supporting values, it was inevitable that the early attempts to bring the issue of management on to the policy agenda foundered on the implacable political logic of this argument. Thus, for example, the report *Management arrangements for the reorganised Health Service* which heralded the management reorganisation of 1974 stated

> The distinguishing characteristic of the NHS is that to do their work properly consultants and general practitioners must have clinical autonomy, so that they can be fully responsible for the treatment they prescribe to their patients. It follows that these doctors and dentists work as each other's equals and that *they are their own managers*. In ethics and law they are accountable to their patients for the care they prescribe and *they cannot be held accountable to the NHS authorities* for the quality of their clinical judgements so long as they act within the broad limits of acceptable medical practice and within policy for the use of resources. (Department of Health and Social Security, 1972: para 1.18; quoted by Stacey, 1984: 13, emphasis added)

In such a situation, administrators acting in support of medical decision-making was the most appropriate form of organisation, reflected in parallel administrative and medical hierarchies extending beyond the individual organisation to the national level. With the reforms of the 1970s, this evolved into what was known as 'consensus management' working through district management teams representing, primarily, medical, administrative and nursing heads (Hunter, 1984).

In the early 1980s, the perennial NHS problem of patient demand outstripping the available supply of health care coupled with the arrival of a confident and radical Conservative government led to a reappraisal of the nature of the high level bargain between medicine and state and consequently of the policy options available. A new view emerged: the traditional mode of informal rationing by the autonomous clinician should be replaced by the explicit management of health care resources in order to improve the efficiency and effectiveness with which health care is delivered. As formally unveiled in the 1983 Griffiths Report, the new policy had two main implications for the medical profession. First, doctors 'must accept the management responsibility which goes with clinical freedom' and take account of the resources which are dispensed as a result of their clinical decisions (Department of Health and Social Security, 1983a: 19). Second, to drive the various initiatives which grew out of the policy, establish a cost-conscious environment and provide greater direction to the management of hospitals, doctors found themselves joined by a new class of general managers. So in terms of policy ambition at least, not only was clinical freedom to be diminished but also a new, state-sponsored power group was in position to promote the linkage between clinical decision making and fixed budgets. As players in the great NHS game, managers had arrived.

Unfortunately, they found themselves deposited by an optimistic state in territory where the natives, if not overtly hostile, were not particularly welcoming either. There was after all no good reason why the medical profession should cooperate either with the policy or with the managers charged with delivering it since there was every chance that, if implemented, the policy would alter the nature of doctors' professional autonomy within the NHS. Once this elementary political fact became apparent and because the profession was too powerful to be told what to do, the DHSS resorted to persuasion and attempted seduction – in the event, neither of which worked. Attempts were made throughout the 1980s to facilitate the implementation of the Griffiths recommendations through the Management Budgeting and Resource Management initiatives which aimed to provide clinicians with computerised financial data systems to aid their decision making, but the interest of clinicians remained largely unengaged. In 1986 the Department of Health and Social Security (DHSS) review of Management Budgeting concluded that it had failed principally through concentrating overmuch on the technical aspects of budgeting at the expense of winning the support and commitment of key personnel: managers, clinicians and finance officers (Young, 1986). So, Resource Management was introduced in its stead as a supposedly wider approach that would emphasise 'medical and nursing ownership of the system' and would generate extensive clinical as well as financial information (Department of Health and Social Security, 1986). But this also proved to be a white elephant.

The use of information systems as a device to tempt clinicians into the parlour of managerial responsibility was always bound to fail because it was not accompanied by incentives to offset the disadvantages to doctors of making such a move. In their study of general management, Harrison and his colleagues observed, whilst quoting a senior hospital doctor, that 'the idea that many clinicians would be interested in taking on time consuming management posts was "one of the serious fallacies of Griffiths"' (Harrison *et al.*, 1989: 11). In part, the shift to Resource Management recognised this issue but since the suggested solutions were more training or an unspecified organisational or cultural change this was scarcely the kind of realism to counter the advantages of money, status and power already enjoyed by doctors (Packwood *et al.*, 1990). Of those who ventured into the field of general management itself, most decided it was not for them. Between 1985 and 1991 the number of doctors heading the management of districts and hospitals halved from 120 to 58. Lack of remuneration is cited as one reason, the loss of private practice and the hostility of medical colleagues as others (Millar, 1991).

While doctors could choose whether or not they engaged with the post-Griffiths drive to improve efficiency in the NHS, the new cadre of general managers enjoyed no such luxury. They were accountable not only for their own performance but also for that of the organisation as a whole; and it was largely the resource allocating decisions of clinicians that determined the latter. General managers were thus in the paradoxical position where they were held accountable for the aggregate decisions of a group (doctors) whose professional ideology, founded on a historic concordat with the state, insisted that its members should only be accountable to each other, if at all, and certainly not to managers. The effect was to give managers considerable responsibility but little power to enable them to progress from the myth of management to its reality.

The political ambiguity of management: secondary care

Writing in 1990, Klein argued that despite the advent of general management little had changed in the relationship between the state and the medical profession since the inception of the NHS: the government sets an overall budget for the Health Service and in turn 'the NHS provides a setting where doctors can exercise their skills with almost complete autonomy' (Klein, 1990: 700). This being the case, we need to reflect on what forces were, and perhaps are, sustaining the position of managers as the chosen vehicle for the state's policy ambitions despite their obvious limitations as a power group. By the late 1980s, the political ambiguity of the managerial role was manifest. Managers were both an established and an ineffectual feature of the NHS: an integral part of the state's approach to health policy yet tolerated by doctors precisely because they wielded little influence.

Two ideological streams converged to give credibility to managers as players in the Health Service and to legitimise their presence on the policy agenda regardless of their political efficacy. First, the New Right developed a view of health care provision which emphasised the importance of consumer choice, the elimination of professional barriers to the operation of the market, and positive public management in the delivery of health care (see Chapter 3). As a strong and continuing influence on Conservative government policy making, such values portrayed managers as an essential component of a consumer-oriented NHS. At the same time, the rise of the New Public Management (NPM) in government sought to change the bureaucratic principles on which the delivery of public services had traditionally rested and to import the managerial values and business techniques of the private sector. Resonating strongly with aspects of the New Right's ideological platform, the NPM advocated an approach to public services characterised by a system of devolved management, responsive to consumer pressure, and capable of utilising market mechanisms within an overall structure of contractual accountability (Ferlie *et al.*, 1996; Hood, 1991; Pollitt, 1990). This new model of the public service is conceived as comprising three elements: 'the corporate core responsible for strategy and policy making; the client side for services, responsible for setting and monitoring standards; and the service provider, who actually delivers services' (Walsh, 1995: 197). Under the new regime, the intention is that the efficient use of public resources will be maximised as a result of their rational disposal by the new class of public service managers. Scientific management becomes the philosopher's stone of modern government and the existing values of service delivery must necessarily adapt or perish. In the managerial cosmos, the values of professional judgement based on trust and status are replaced by contractual relations driven by the 'objective' analysis of client needs.

The impact of the new management values on the formal fabric of the public services has been substantial. Reforms such as those driven by the Next Steps Initiative, the Financial Management Initiative and market testing have aimed to reconfigure radically the structures through which the state fulfils its responsibilities to its citizens (Giddings, 1995; Walsh, 1995). However, whilst the incorporation of such reforms into an institutional culture could proceed reasonably smoothly in uncontroversial areas such as vehicle licensing, in the highly politicised and idiosyncratic environment of the NHS, thickly populated by a dense jungle of dispersed medical powers, the progress of the managerial mission was bound to be slow.

Nonetheless, by the late 1980s the twin ideological themes of market and management were a central tenet in government policy making. Flanked by a burgeoning group of academics to reflect on how policy should be formed and an array of management consultants to help implement it, the government had no doubts about the value of the new creed. If managers had yet to make an impact in the Health Service then this must be because they lacked the appropriate policy to release their potential. It was significant that in formulating such a policy in the course of the 1989 Review of the NHS, the state chose this moment to abandon its long established corporatist agreement with medicine. Henceforth, the 'iron triangle' of the medical profession, officials and ministers was, it seemed, to be consigned to the dustbin of history and the profession excluded from the inner policy community (Butler, 1992; Haywood and Hunter, 1982).

The subsequent White Paper *Working for patients* and the 1990 NHS and Community Care Act established a new organisational framework for the Health Service based on the concept of an internal market in the NHS: a division between the purchasers and providers of health care, competition between providers, devolved operational management, and a continuing drive towards greater efficiency (Department of Health, 1989a). Within the new policy, managers were accorded a pivotal implementation role. They were the change agents who would relieve the political pressure on the state by providing citizens with the Health Service they expected. Rather than the covert rationing of citizen demand by clinicians, the state could expect to rely on the efficient management of health care supply by managers. With the introduction of the internal market policy, managers were intended to replace doctors as the primary functionaries in the delivery of citizens' health care rights and, thereby, to diminish, if not remove, the state's dependence on medicine in its relationship with civil society. How was this to be achieved?

Working for patients describes how NHS Hospital Trusts were to have a range of powers and freedoms not available to the then existing District Health Authorities (DHAs).

NHS Hospital Trusts will be empowered by statute to employ staff; to enter into contracts both to provide services and to buy in services and supplies with others; and to raise income within the scope set by the Health and Medicine's Act 1988. (Department of Health, 1989a: 23)

Trust activity, and therefore the activity of their doctors, was to be determined by the services contracted from them by DHAs engaged in purchasing the health care required to meet the needs of the local population. The tradition of 'producer capture' of the Health Service by the medical profession was to be replaced by a needs-driven approach which would make the service more responsive to patients. As far as the key actors in the new scenario were concerned, *Working for patients* was clear that its proposals were building on the general management structures already established (Department of Health, 1989a: 11). These would be used 'to ensure that consultants are properly accountable for the consequences of [their] decisions', that medical audit was appropriately developed, and that the consultant's job contract and distinction awards (once reformed) were suitably managed (Department of Health, 1989a: Chapter 5). In terms of formal policy intent, NHS managers were in pole position.

Given the managerial ambitions of the internal market policy, it is instructive to follow through the logic of its organisational implementation. How, exactly, were managers going to manage doctors? In secondary care, responsibility for ensuring the delivery of the health care contracts purchased by the DHAs rested with the chief executive and the Trust Board to whom led all the lines of accountability in the organisation. Following the Griffiths Report, there had been much debate about the appropriate organisational unit to facilitate the linkage between clinical decisions and resource allocation. The favoured model which emerged was that of the clinical directorate: a semi-autonomous unit, based on a medical specialty or group of specialties, usually managed by a clinician, to which full budgetary responsibility is devolved and within which the Griffiths objective of combining clinical and budgetary decision could be achieved (BMA Central Consultants and Specialists Committee, 1990; Institute of Health Services Management, 1990). The optimistic managerial assumption was that the clinical directorate would make it possible 'to overlay the medical staff organisation on the management hierarchies' and so achieve 'an organisational bonding' between these hitherto separate entities (Institute of Health Services Management, 1990: 5).

In terms of the managerial details of the clinical directorate's operation, it was commonly accepted that its clinical management team should be composed of a clinical director, senior nurse manager and business manager; but there was less agreement on the distribution of responsibilities and powers and who was to be held accountable for coordinating which aspects of the directorate's work. Although it was generally assumed that the clinical director should be a clinician in order to be able to command respect from senior or junior doctors, there remained the thorny problem that respect is not necessarily the same thing as authority. In his account of how Guy's Hospital dealt with the issue of clinical leadership, a senior member of the medical profession observed that 'all consultants in the NHS have equal status and the possibility that any one of them should have authority over others is properly resisted' (Chantler, 1990). His solution was for authority to rest with a group of clinicians with a clinical director taking responsibility for the provision of service, a somewhat unwieldy device, particularly in the not unknown situation where there are disputes about the allocation of scarce resources.

Even if the issues of role division and clinical director authority were resolved, there remained the problem of the motivation of the clinician in management. Still unaddressed were the financial and career incentives required to facilitate the integration of the clinical directorate within a contract driven framework of management (Spry, 1990: 10). In the early 1990s, within the distinction award system of salary supplements for clinicians, only the lowest category of award included management responsibility as one of its criteria and it is doubtful whether this was a significant factor in the decision, dominated as the procedure was by the clinicians themselves. From the beginning, Trusts made specific payments to clinical directors for taking on this management role but these were usually too small to act as a serious incentive and insufficient to offset the loss of the clinician's private practice which frequently accompanied the new responsibilities (British Association of Medical Managers et al., 1993: 30). Specialties varied in the extent to which they engaged with the management requirements of the new policy. Historically, the diagnostic and support directorates of pharmacy, pathology and radiology have been delegated considerable budgetary and decision-making powers and were therefore more responsive (Grossman, 1990: 13; Institute of Health Services Management, 1990: 6). Nonetheless, the phenomenon of the reluctant clinical director was the pervasive one (Salter, 1994: 66–8).

Not surprisingly, therefore, the adoption of the clinical directorate model as the means for engaging hospital clinicians in management was a slow process. In 1990, 40 per cent of hospital units had clinical directorates whilst 80 per cent had at least some clinicians holding budgets (Tomlin, 1990). Three years later, a survey conducted by the British Association of Medical Managers revealed a mixed picture. Most providing organisations were found to have a decentralised clinical management structure based on clinical groupings but the proportion of the total unit budget actually devolved to these groupings ranged from under 10 per cent to over 90 per cent with an average of between 50 and 70 per cent (British Association of Medical Managers *et al.*, 1993: 18).

The partial and often reluctant involvement of the clinician in management was a shaky platform on which to build a policy as ambitious and radical as that of the internal market. As the 1991 reforms increased the intensity and specificity of the contract-based cost pressures on Trusts, so hospital managers were given the responsibility of ensuring that the clinical priorities of clinicians were adapted to their organisations' contractual needs – with or without the cooperation of clinical directors. What levers did they possess to launch such a direct confrontation with the principle of clinical autonomy? It was one of the cardinal freedoms of Trust that they would be able to employ staff on the conditions they considered appropriate and pay them what they chose (Department of Health, 1989a: 25, 1989b). In line with this policy, consultant employment contracts were transferred from Regional Health Authorities (RHAs) to Trusts and chief executives were made full members of the Advisory Appointments Committees for consultants which nonetheless continued to be professionally dominated (National Health Service Management Executive, 1991a). The intention was also 'to introduce arrangements which will more clearly define the scope and extent of each consultant's duties' through a job description which would include hours worked, medical audit, budgetary and management responsibilities and an annual review (Department of Health, 1989b: 5–6). Apparently, procedures were to be put in place which would enable managers to bring doctors into the mainstream of Trusts' accountability systems.

For a time it was possible for official voices to sustain the myth that statements of procedural intent would be followed by a consequent shift in the power relationship between doctors and managers and that the latter were still driving policy forward. Thus, for example, we find the Audit Commission in a 1994 report conflating intention with effect:

> Managers now have more control over the employment of staff and the management of capital. They have taken over the employment of consultants from regional or district health authorities and they can negotiate local pay and conditions for a wide range of staff. They can use retained surpluses or Treasury capital within their external financing

limit and they can enter into arrangements that use private sector capital such as operating leases or joint ventures, provided the risk is equitably shared. And it is now more acceptable to consider sub-contracting services, leaving managers free to concentrate on core activities. (Audit Commission, 1994: 3)

In reality, research has shown that doctors' influence during this period remained largely undiminished (Harrison *et al.*, 1992). As Harrison and Pollitt observe 'it seems that doctors retained a good deal of *covert* influence; many general managers expected doctors to be difficult, and therefore refrained from raising issues that might arouse opposition, preferring instead to leave matters to be dealt with by peer pressure' (Harrison and Pollitt, 1994: 50). Medical audit, for example, remained the province of doctors, relied exclusively on peer review, was often carried out on a local and unsystematic basis, and results were often not shared or disseminated (Kerrison *et al.*, 1993; Pollitt, 1993).

That managers should have been reticent about confronting doctors is not surprising. Managers were a relatively new power group in NHS politics, propelled to the sharp end of policy implementation by politicians with their customary expectations about quick results, yet required to deal with an established professional body with many and varied sources of power. As they engaged with doctors, managers had to bear in mind their employment situation. Whereas hospital doctors were, and are, protected by an array of professional defences which heavily dilute the effectiveness of employment and disciplinary sanctions, managers were usually appointed on short-term contracts which inevitably heightened their exposure to the pressures from their political masters. Trust chief executives and chairs were no more protected than were junior managers, perhaps less so since the accountability arrangements from above and below tended to focus on their roles. Should clinicians decide to go public in their dispute with senior management, there was usually only one outcome. As John Spiers, who as chair of Brighton Health Care Trust in 1994 was obliged to resign following a vote of no confidence from his consultants, observed: 'When I speak to managers around the country the message I hear is the same. They say: "Look what happened to you in Brighton – we don't dare take them [the clinicians] on"' (Waters, 1995: 13).

As managers dutifully sought to pursue the logic of the 1991 reforms, so the fundamental collision between the managerial and clinical cultures became manifest and the space for the exercise of mutual tolerance shrank rapidly. As Hunter observes, the basic difference is a simple one: 'The concern of doctors to do what is best for the individual patient may conflict with the need [of managers] to set priorities within services, to maintain expenditure within agreed limits, and to maximise the benefits of service to the population served' (Hunter, 1991: 443). Legitimised by the principle of clinical freedom, the medical focus on the patient interest at the exclusion of all others leads in its pure form to a rejection of any involvement in management since this could compromise the exercise of clinical judgement (Chant, 1984). That this was a common view at the time of the internal market policy is substantiated by a National Health Service Executive (NHSE) survey in 1995 which found that 70 per cent of doctors rejected management as part of their everyday clinical practice (Turner, 1995: 13). The two opposing cultures effectively created two organisations in one which, when subject to contract driven demands, viewed each other with mutual hostility. From being tolerated by doctors in the immediate post-Griffiths era, with the implementation of *Working for patients* managers found themselves regarded with suspicion and labelled as the agents of the state – which of course they were (Dawson, 1994).

A management vacuum: primary care

Despite the rhetoric of devolved operational management, the centralised accountability systems introduced by the internal market reforms ensured that local NHS managers in secondary care had little freedom of manoeuvre as they struggled to meet both the agendas of purchasing agencies and the national targets of the Patients Charter. Caught between the rock of their contractual obligations and the hard place of medical autonomy, managers were obliged to deal with their powerlessness through the constructive use of political ambiguity.

In primary care, where over a third of the medical profession reside, the relationship between doctors and managers has been much less confined and the challenge to medical power at best diffuse. Until 1990 when the Family Health Services Authorities (FHSAs) were introduced, the NHS bureaucracy of primary care never pretended to be anything other than a vehicle for passively channelling funds according to a national formula to the small businesses of independent GPs. Its budget was calculated and administered separately from that of the rest of the NHS: from 1948 to 1974 through executive councils and from 1974 to 1990 by Family Practitioner Committees (FPCs). Their upward lines of accountability ran directly to the Department of Health, bypassing the RHAs with their planning and management machinery, and were never politicised to the same degree as those in the acute sector. The Griffiths Report and the general management enthusiasms of the 1980s left the FPCs largely unmoved; not surprisingly given that 90 per cent of their budget was demand led, not cash limited, and largely uncontrollable (Audit Commission, 1993: 52). Even the numbers and distribution of GPs were outside the remit of the state bureaucracy, being determined by the professionally dominated Medical Practices Committee.

At the end of the 1980s, and like their colleagues in secondary care, GPs found themselves subject to two types of pressures to deal with the disjunction between patient demand and primary care supply: first, accountability to a new class of managers and, second, self-management of the relationship between clinical activity and the resources available. The attempt at direct managerial intervention began in April 1990 when the new GP Contract was introduced in the teeth of opposition from the medical profession. It constituted a clear ambition to provide the new FHSAs with a management tool in their dealings with GPs. The Contract changed the make up of GPs' incomes by increasing the proportion of that income determined by the numbers of people on doctors' lists ('capitation fees') and by introducing a system of performance-related payments linked to the provision of specific primary care services such as health promotion clinics, immunisation and screening targets, and minor surgery. However, whether the new FHSAs would have the capacity to activate and implement this management potential was another matter.

Superficially, they were different organisational animals from their FPC predecessors. The NHS and Community Care Act 1990 had streamlined their structure, introduced general management, given them responsibility for ensuring medical audit was carried out by GPs, and placed prescribing costs within a fixed FHSA budget administered through a system of indicative pre-scribing (Department of Health, 1989a: 56–8). The latter was the most significant departure from previous practice because for the first time a core part of GP expenditure was, in theory at least, made cash limited. It constituted a direct response to the increase in NHS drugs expenditure (of which GP prescribing was the largest part) of 4 per cent per year above the rate of inflation in the 5 years up to the publication of *Working for patients*. Cash limited budgets were also introduced for improvements to GP premises and the staffing of primary care team members directly employed by the practice (Department of Health, 1989c: 6).

As in secondary care, the attempted implementation of these reforms was accompanied by a self-deceiving official rhetoric which equated organisational re-labelling and new paper functions with genuine power shifts between doctors and managers. Thus Andrew Foster, then deputy chief executive of the NHS, observed that the remarkable degree of autonomy previously enjoyed by independent GP practitioners was being challenged by the new breed of FHSA general managers. He continued:

> the developments of 1990 began to establish the FHS as a managed public service with GPs held responsible for the provision of specified information, and of hours, times and types of service that would have been unthinkable just a few years ago. Existing boundaries between the clinical and the managerial have been tested and have begun to move. (Foster, 1991: 8)

Similarly, in the same year the National Health Service Management Executive (NHSME)'s *Integrating primary and secondary health care* claimed that the new GP Contract 'has already shown itself to be a powerful instrument for strategic change in the NHS' and argued that FHSAs should be given greater discretion in manag-ing the Contract to enable them to target efforts and resources on those practices and patients where there is greatest need (National Health Service Management Executive, 1991b: 2–3).

While such statements may have been a useful expression of senior management ideology and self-belief, they bore little relation-ship to the difficulties of changing the traditional, and largely passive, administration of the FPCs into an efficient FHSA management tool for dealing with entrenched medical power. In the early 1990s, the FHSA budget was a product of historical patterns of expenditure, largely unrelated to population characteristics, and therefore not compatible with the policy rhetoric of the time regarding the needs based approach of NHS planning and management. Nor did they possess the capacity for the directed expenditure of the budget for which they were responsible. With the FHS budget category, 90 per cent of General Medical Services (GMS) expenditure (payments for services to patients, capitation payments for GP lists, drugs prescribed) was not controlled by the FHSA but driven by the demand from GPs who did not regard their activities as cash limited (Audit Commission, 1993: 11). Most of the 10 per cent balance of GMS expenditure where the FHSA did exercise control and which was cash limited (computers, practice premises, practice staff) was in any case committed in advance.

In embarking on their chosen mission of bringing GPs within the orbit of management control, FHSAs were therefore starting from a very low management base as they engaged with independent practitioners unused and unsympathetic to most forms of external bureaucratic accountability. In the area of prescribing, for example, the government's formal ambition was 'to place downward pressure on expenditure on drugs in order to eliminate waste and to release resources for other parts of the health service' (Department of Health, 1989d: 3). The chosen mechanism was indicative prescribing which, building on the Prescribing Analysis and Cost (PACT) system of self-audit by GPs, gave FHSAs the task of monitoring practice drug expenditure against a fixed target on a monthly basis. However, regardless of NHSME managerial rhetoric, the whole exercise was still dependent on the goodwill of independent GPs because there was no sanction which could be used against them if they felt disinclined to cooperate.

Lacking both capacity and power, FHSA managers were in no position to use the 1990 Contract as a vehicle for redefining their relationship with general practitioners. Instead, and given the absence of managerial control, the implementation of the Contract was propelled by the forces of individual clinical autonomy, as primary care in general had always been. The Contract therefore acted as a set of financial incentives for GPs to expand the range of services they provided according to their individual interests and perceptions of patient need which, in aggregate, produced a random effect. Existing health promotion clinics increased their activity, new ones were established (e.g. asthma and diabetes) and GPs paid great attention to reaching their immunisation and cervical cytology targets (Leese and Bosanquet, 1995). There was wide variation between practices in their uptake of the incentives and little relationship between the provision of new services and any managerially defined view of the health care needs of the local population. Indeed, the reverse might happen because there was the strong possibility, as Hopton and Dlugolecka observe, that by 'encouraging a focus on particular areas of care, national policy may lead to a relative neglect of greater need in areas not linked to financial incentives' (Hopton and Dlugolecka, 1995: 1372).

Although the introduction of general management in primary care had little observable effect on the autonomy of doctors in that sector, a second policy initiative within the 1990 reforms which aimed at introducing a new form of cash limited self-management by GPs initially seemed to offer a more sophisticated way of restricting the clinical freedoms of this part of the medical profession. Like Management Budgeting, Resource Management and the role of clinical director in secondary, GP Fundholding sought to place doctors in the position where they were obliged to accept responsibility for managing the relationship between patient demand for health care and the available supply. However, unlike their medical colleagues in the acute sector, GPs who signed up to the Fundholding scheme which commenced on 1 April 1991 were asked to carry out this rationing activity through both a providing and a purchasing function. On the provider side, the Fundholder budget included two aspects of GP primary care services: 70 per cent of practice team staff costs, and, most importantly, prescribing. On the purchaser side, it included three categories of hospital services: outpatients, a defined group of inpatient and day case treatments and diagnostic tests. Fundholders were also given a fee to cover the management and other costs of participating in the scheme (Department of Health, 1989a: 49, 1989e). Most importantly, each Fundholder budget was cash limited though virement was allowed between the different categories of Fundholder expenditure. Separate to this budget was the normal GP Contract with the FHSA for the provision of the remaining categories of primary care services.

Given that the ambition of the Fundholder policy was clearly to circumscribe the clinical freedom of general practitioners by ensuring that both their providing decisions (the supply of primary care) and their purchasing decisions (the demand for secondary care) were restricted by the requirement to work within a fixed Fundholder budget, why did doctors agree to take on what had previously been a political responsibility of the state? It has to be remembered that although general practice is regarded as part of the NHS it is, along with dental practice, ophthalmology and pharmacy, first and foremost a collection of small businesses which contract with the Health Service to provide a primary care service. Given that the financial health of the practice had always been a central GP concern, this may explain why some GPs took to the idea of a competitive internal market more readily than did NHS managers (Glennerster *et al.*, 1994: 48). For them, Fundholding was a step along a path which enabled them to improve their businesses with little or no cost to themselves. Hence when asked why they joined the scheme, their stated reasons were to improve the quality of the service they provided, the opportunity to have more services on site, greater freedom of referral and budgetary freedoms – familiar business arguments (Glennester *et al.*, 1994: 46).

Nor would potential Fundholders have been unduly troubled by the accountability mechanisms of the new arrangement since these were virtually non-existent and did not constitute a disincentive. The Fundholder budget was to be determined and allocated by the RHAs and monitored by the FHSAs. However, not only was there no contract to structure the relationship between NHS and Fundholder but also, as we have already seen, the capacity of the FHSAs to assume any additional management functions was severely limited. One unusual consequence of this 'management gap' was that the financial regulations allowed Fundholders to retain any audited underspends on their budgets while overspends were to be met by the Health Authority (Audit Commission, 1995a: 19). Health Authorities were encouraged to negotiate the return of underspends but had no powers to support their negotiating intentions. As a result, in 1993–94, three-quarters of Fundholders made a saving (20 per cent of £100 000 or more) and of these about 10 per cent returned part of this underspend. Although Fundholders were theoretically constrained in the disposal of these savings in that they had to be spent in ways which were 'for the benefit of the patients of the practice', since this could include improvements to the practice premises (and hence the market value of the business property) the incentives to underspend were obvious (Audit Commission, 1996a: 72). It is impossible to conceive that any other group in the private sector of health care could have negotiated such a favourable financial relationship with the NHS.

Interestingly, it was probably in terms of the purchasing function that the managerial potential of Fundholding was most fully realised. Rather than bringing doctors within the orbit of managers, the effect of Fundholders as purchasers was to bring doctors (consultants) within the managerial orbit of other doctors (GPs). In so doing, Fundholding acted more to stimulate (albeit short-lived) changes in the medical profession than it did to impose a managerial discipline on general practitioners themselves. For, Fundholding held out to GPs the prospect that by acting as the agents of the state in the contracting of secondary care, they could re-engineer the status and power differences between themselves and hospital doctors. Historically, GPs had never been able to realise the potential advantage embodied in their exclusive power of referral because, for practical and professional reasons, they had needed hospital specialists more than specialists had needed them. Once a GP referral was made, a patient's subsequent progress through the outpatient waiting list, the outpatient treatment, the in- or day-patient waiting list, the in- or day-patient treatment, and discharge back to the GP was wholly controlled by the hospital consultant. GPs might murmur about waiting times of dilatory discharge letters but their professional subordination meant they could not challenge.

Fundholding challenged the traditional assumptions of this relationship and gave GPs the financial and contractual muscle to hold their consultant colleagues to account for the quantity and quality of health care provided in terms of, for example, waiting times for patient appointments, standards of care, and the speed at which discharge letters were received (Glennerster *et al.*, 1994: 68–70). Some parts of the hospital service, and some consultants, were more responsive than others to the potential loss of GP Fundholder income and the reordering of the medical hierarchy which responsiveness entailed. Where consultants proved to be reluctant converts to the new way of doing things, the interesting situation could arise of hospital managers being obliged to act on behalf of Fundholder doctors in order to bring hospital doctors into line with a Fundholder's contractual requirements.

Following the entry of the first wave of about 300 practices into the scheme in 1991, the numbers grew quickly and by April 1996 had reached about 2200 covering about half the population (Audit Commission, 1996a: 8). In April 1993, the BMA abandoned its opposition to the scheme and the stage was set for the state to consolidate and expand the power of its chosen professional allies. The extension of the Fundholder scheme in April 1993 pursued the natural logic of the GP-centred primary health care team and, in so doing, achieved a substantial redistribution of financial power to general practitioners. From within the Hospital and Community Health Services (HCHS) budget as a whole, Fundholders were given all the non-acute elements of the community health services budget (community nursing, paramedical services, specialist nursing); the mental illness budget (day case, outpatients, community); and the learning disability budget (outpatients, community) (Audit Commission, 1995a: appendix 1). Under the cover of extending an existing policy, the boundaries between primary and secondary care were redrawn and whole groups of health care professionals (e.g. district nurses, health visitors, community psychiatric nurses) transferred to the GP Fundholders' sphere of influence.

In facilitating this transfer of financial and decision-making power to a private sector group of medical professionals, the state was clearly taking a political risk. The logic of the professional solution to the supply–demand mismatch in health care assumes that clinical judgement is used to manage demand by tailoring it to fit the available supply. It is a supply-led solution where the doctor accepts a fixed budget as the framework for the management activity. However, the budgetary basis of the scheme undermined this logic from the beginning because Fundholding GPs received two budgets, one of which was fixed (the Fundholding budget) and the other open ended (the GP Contract). While the former pursed the path of the supply-led solution with its built in rationing assumptions, the latter was demand led, non-rationing and characterised by task-driven incentives which encouraged the expansion of health care demand in areas such as health promotion. Further confusion arose from the fact that there was no simple functional divide between the activities funded by the two budgets: thus through its prescribing and community health service elements, the Fundholding budget incorporated primary provision as well as the secondary care purchasing function. So, Fundholders found themselves subject to different self-management pressures as a result of the contradictory implications of rationing and non-rationing behaviour.

With the 1996 NHS Act, FHSAs were merged with DHAs to form the new unitary Health Authorities which then took up responsibility for the monitoring of Fundholders. Significantly, the total cost of Fundholding for a given Health Authority became part of that Authority's cash limited budget for which it was responsible through its corporate contract with the NHSE. If Fundholders overspent, as they were allowed to do, and if this meant that the Health Authority as a whole overspent, this would be regarded as management failure on the part of the Authority and penalised accordingly. There were therefore strong inducements for Health Authorities to develop a management capacity to improve the very loose accountability arrangements under which GP Fundholders had this far operated. Unlike FHSAs, Health Authorities had at least some management resources with which to undertake this task. Unfortunately, given the state's commitment to the professional autonomy of GPs as a condition of their involvement in the Fundholder policy, the central guidance on the appropriate forms of accountability to be introduced was, perhaps inevitably, very bland and left Health Authority managers once again in an ambiguous position. They were advised that as general practitioners became increasingly important as purchasers 'Health Authorities needed to shift the balance of their activity towards these strategic, monitoring and support [of GPs] roles' (National Health Service Executive, 1994a: 2). When translated into 'principles of accountability' the situation remained equally ill defined.

> Health Authorities have statutory responsibility for *leading* the implementation of Government policy at local level. This includes *advising* and *informing* GP fundholders of the wider implications of their purchasing intentions (such as the impact on hospitals or community units or on local strategy) but without second-guessing clinical and management decisions taken by GPs on behalf of their patients. (National Health Service Executive, 1994b: 3, emphases added)

This is scarcely the language of self-confident management. In any case, given that Fundholders' statutory accountability was direct to the NHSE via its regional offices, and not to Health Authorities, the latter lacked the formal powers to enforce any accountability procedures it might put in place.

Conclusions

The policy experience of GP Fundholding nicely encapsulates one of the central dilemmas faced by the state in its dealings with the medical profession. It may begin with high hopes of engineering a significant change in the delivery of health care, enact a raft of radical legislative measures, redesign structures and create a high profile role for managers as agents in the change process. But ultimately the ability to implement policy in the NHS will depend on the cooperation of the dominant power group: the doctors. The internal market reforms began with managers apparently at the policy wheel in the secondary sector, yet from the outset in primary care the managerial vacuum was so inescapable that GPs had, of necessity, to be in the driving seat. This gave them a pivotal bargaining position from which much flowed.

By the end of the 1980s, the difficulties experienced in the introduction of general management following the Griffiths Report had already shown that the medical profession was, at best, indifferent and, at worst, implacably hostile to any managerial challenge to its traditional hegemony in the NHS. Similarly, policies aimed at persuading clinicians that they should themselves take on the mantle of squaring the circle between finite public resources for health care and an ever expanding demand from citizens had received an unenthusiastic response. Some hospitals had begun to introduce clinical directorates as an organisational vehicle for the involvement of doctors in management but progress was slow. Meanwhile the high level concordat between medicine and the state which had underpinned the policy-making process since the inception of the Health Service in 1948 had, to all intents and purposes, dissolved.

Given the clear limitations of the general management policy, there is a need to explain why the Conservative government was so optimistic regarding the implementation of the 1990 reforms, so convinced of the contribution that managers would make to this process and so unaware, apparently, of the consequences of excluding the medical profession from the policy-making process during the 1989 Review. In part, the explanation may lie in the political impetus generated by the New Public Management as a self-confident style of bureaucratic governance and the ideological impetus embodied in the New Right's influence on Conservative Party thinking. Together they mobilised a policy momentum which placed Health Service managers at the forefront of the proposed changes. Furthermore, when it came to the details of the managerial implementation of these changes, *Working for patients* and its many supporting policy documents displayed characteristics which, as Stewart has noted of the NPM approach in general, serve to foster a false optimism:

> generally there is a tendency to simplify management tasks in the belief that clear targets and separation of roles can clarify responsibility and release management initiative. Simplification has been achieved by the separation of policy from implementation, the development of contracts, quasi-contracts or targets governing relationships, and their enforcement by performance management. (Stewart, 1998: 16)

Instead, he and Ranson argue, 'a concept of management is needed which encompasses the recognition of political difference and conflict as constitutive of a public organisation rather than an obstacle to it' (Ranson and Stewart, 1989: 5–6). Just because an organisation is defined in managerial terms does not mean that it is thereby depoliticised.

The failure of policy makers to consider policy implementation as anything other than a process of rationalistic, goal-oriented management left the NHS managers of the early and mid-1990s in an exposed position. They were expected by politicians to deliver a policy but lacked the political tools with which to do it. Doctors, as the power group *in situ* with no ownership of the internal market policy, were bound to resist. To deal with this opposition, managers focused on the redefinition and the relabelling of structures, some redirection of the flows of money between organisations and units through the new purchasing function, and efforts at cost-containment. These were feeble instruments, for two reasons. First, the GP Fundholder scheme instituted a counter financial dynamic controlled by doctors not managers. Second, clinical activity, the arena where all meaningful decisions about the relationship between the supply of and demand for health care were made, remained the sole province of the medical profession. As a result, the allocations of finance continued to follow the medical definition of patient need. For their part, few hospital doctors perceived financial or managerial concerns as affecting their practice as a result of the reforms; and of those involved in management, clinical directors and medical directors continued to identify themselves as professionals rather than managers (Sutherland and Dawson, 1998: S20). Indeed, clinical directors can be seen as having remained professionals but with added power as a result of the reforms. Likewise, in primary care GP Fundholders increased their economic autonomy through an extension of the financial arenas under their control.

The 1990 reforms gave managers influence over the context within which doctors worked but not over the clinical activity itself. Regulation of what doctors did, how they did it, how judgements were made about the quality of their performance, and what corrective sanctions, if any, should be taken remained almost wholly within the medical domain. Ultimately, doctors would cooperate with managerial objectives if they chose to, or if enough of their colleagues chose to. Unlike managers, they were not politically dispensable.

The political vulnerability of managers increased as their inability to implement the cost limiting ambitions of the internal market policy became manifest. In April 1994, the then Secretary of State for Health, Virginia Bottomley, responding to Labour Party criticism of the burgeoning bureaucracy of the internal market, launched a drive to identify the management costs of Trusts. In its report on the subject, which showed the wide variation in Trusts' management costs, the Audit Commission duly warned, in barbed tones, that to 'constrain or even reduce management expenditure in the absence of any evidence on what benefits it does or does not achieve, is a dangerous game, however popular it might make the player' (Audit Commission, 1995b: 14). However, since popularity is a key measure of political success it was therefore perfectly natural that in 1996 Mrs Bottomley's successor, Steven Dorrell, should demand a 5 per cent across the board reduction in Trusts' management spending emphasising the importance of 'white coats over grey suits'.

As managers moved seamlessly from change agents to political scapegoats (a role they were to retain for future use), so the attempt by the state to reduce its dependence on medicine for the delivery of citizens' health care rights duly faded. The medical profession, for its part, had also had time to reconsider its position. Having been coldshouldered and marginalised during the 1989 Review of the NHS it too was reflecting on the need to minimise conflict with the state and regain its customary access to the inner circle of the health policy community. Both were aware of the advantages of a new definition of the historic concordat. But with the victory of the Labour Party in the 1997 election, a fresh dynamic was to enter the political stage.

5

The parallel world of medicine

Introduction

Much of NHS policy is based on the erroneous assumption that managers have the ability to implement it. As Chapter 4 has shown and Chapter 6 will illuminate through an account of political drama, that ability is severely constrained by the need to recruit the support of those who mainly dispose of NHS resources: the doctors. Should doctors decide not to cooperate, or to cooperate only partially, Health Service managers are obliged to spin dream-webs of apparent progress to assuage the wrath of their frustrated political leaders. Given the historic bargain between medicine and the state of which professional self-regulation is the single most powerful expression, managers lack the means to enforce their will on the NHS organisations for which they are responsible.

But what, exactly, is the nature of the political world of medicine which is so impervious to the policy ambitions of the state? How is it maintained and what is the engagement between its different parts? In answering these questions it is important to recall that the profession's power is derived from its regulation of medical knowledge in the arenas of its creation (research), transmission (education), and application (performance) (Table 1.1) – all else flows from this primary source. Over time, British medicine has constructed a labyrinth of roles, rules, procedures and institutions to govern itself through its knowledge-control functions. It is a state within a state, a life-world with its own values, hierarchies and embedded understandings. With the creation of the NHS in 1948 certain accommodations were made between the world of medicine and that of the Health Service. But at no point did the profession relinquish its grip on the regulation of its knowledge. Rather, it ensured that the organisational contours of the NHS were shaped around the outlines of medicine's existing regulatory institutions.

In examining the three regulatory arenas of research, education and performance, this chapter deals not only with the myriad institutions which govern these fields but also with the interconnecting networks which allow power to be diffused across them. For it is a characteristic of medical power that it does not present a single target to any potential state incursion but rather several targets – which can create uncertainty in the mind of the aggressor. Furthermore, regulatory functions are not necessarily neatly divided or uniformly implemented but may rely instead on historic understandings readily accessible to the insiders of the medical elites but much less so to the policy makers of the state.

Research

In order for the legitimacy of medical decisions to be sustained over time, the knowledge base for those decisions has to be seen as both valid and reliable. Up to the early 1970s, it was assumed that no formal mechanism was needed to ensure public trust in medical research and that the values of the profession would naturally guide the individual researcher to square the eternal circle between the interests of the project, the research subject and society. However, Pappworth's seminal work *Human guinea pigs* first published in 1967 cast serious doubt on this assumption by showing that medical researchers not only 'engineered consent' by using a patient's dependency to recruit 'volunteers' but in numerous cases did not obtain consent at all; researchers did not view the ethics of their relationship with their subjects as a salient issue (Pappworth, 1969). Following debates within the profession and recommendations by the Royal College of Physicians on the establishment and composition of Research Ethics Committees (RECs), in 1975 the state duly gave its imprimatur to the proposed addition to medicine's self-regulatory domain by issuing an advisory circular supporting those recommendations (Department of Health and Social Security, 1975). The concordat between medicine and the state was operating in its normal fashion.

As the response to a perceived problem of public trust, the invention of RECs sought to achieve the maximum political gain with the minimum professional disruption. Despite their aura of bureaucratic legitimacy, ethics committees were not introduced as the local components of a national system of research regulation: that is, they were not characterised by common structures, functions, rules and procedures and did not have statutory powers of standard setting, monitoring and intervention. They were advisory not executive bodies. A survey of RECs in England and Wales in 1991 – which included the full range of RECs serving health authority districts, single hospitals, single medical specialties, research institutes and Royal Colleges – established the wide variety that blossomed as a result (Hall, 1991). RECs varied in size from 3 to 41 members with the majority being hospital doctors. In terms of procedures, only 30 per cent of RECs had a standard application form, less than half ever asked for a progress report on approved projects and only 43 per cent ever requested a final report. On the issue of informed consent, and focusing in particular on research on children, the survey reported that 18 per cent of RECs recorded that though they 'usually' or 'sometimes' insisted upon consent, they did not always do so.

Behind these bare statistics lies the evidence of a political compromise which resonated easily with the accepted principles of self-regulation and in no sense conformed to the principles of bureaucratic rationality. Equipped with a majority of medical members, RECs took their authority from their assumed capacity to access and apply the embedded values of medical culture, not from any notion of a bureaucratic legitimacy derived from an accountability to the apparatus of the state. They were also essentially local bodies, shaped by the immediate medical networks and personalities, a product of local medical history. That in an overall sense they grew haphazardly is therefore to be expected since organic institutional adaptation is a central characteristic of medicine's approach to change. They were not an imposition (originally at least) but a regulatory adjunct to the local professional identity. For this reason, it took time for them to develop a specialist identity and to see themselves as possessing and applying a particular ethical expertise. Even in 1991, some fifteen years after the introduction of RECs, fewer than half their members claimed any expertise in ethical judgements (Hall, 1991: 340). Where they did, and where medical ethical expertise forms a distinctive element in REC decision making, it is arguable whether this thus establishes an oppositional dynamic to the medical research interest or whether medical ethics may be, as Stacey has argued, as much about protection of the profession as about protection of the public (Stacey, 1985).

Within the policy discourse of medicine, it is customary to regard lay participation in self-regulation as the formal mechanism for the representation of the public voice. In the case of the regulation of research, as with other forms of professional self-government, that voice has been either weak, non-existent or suspect. Although the 1975 DHSS guidelines recommended that there should be at least 1 lay participant, the 1991 survey showed that 14 per cent of RECs had none (53 per cent had 1 lay member) (Hall, 1991: 337). Perhaps more important is the nature of the lay membership and its ability, or inability, to challenge the medical values which would naturally dominate the REC narrative. A detailed examination of lay members found that 42 per cent would probably not satisfy the requirements of independence made by Federal regulations for Institutional Review Boards (the equivalent of RECs) in the US (Nicholson, 1986). To the extent that lay participation is not independent and to the extent that it is absorbed into the dominant medical discourse of REC discussions, it can be seen in Hall's nice turn of phrase as 'the proxy cooptation of the interests of the research subjects' (Hall, 1991: 337).

As an extension of the territory of medicine, RECs and the research they regulate are protected from external scrutiny by the requirement that they are convened in private, the confidentiality of their proceedings and their very limited reporting responsibilities (Bendall, 1994; Department of Health, 1994b). Formally, local research ethics committees (LRECs) are required to file annual reports to the director of public health of their health authority and multicentre research ethics committees (MRECs) to the Secretary of State for Health (Department of Health, 1991, 1997c). However, the reports contain only minimal information about the studies considered and nothing about the discussions that took place (Foster *et al.*, 1995). Although the responsible authority can ask to see the minutes of REC meetings, they remain confidential documents. In the case of certain types of clinical research funded by pharmaceutical companies, the REC culture of secrecy is reinforced by the need for commercial confidentiality: the Medicines Act 1968 makes it a criminal offence to reveal evidence submitted to, or discussions resulting from, approaches to drugs-regulatory agencies and this may be relevant to phase I clinical trials and other early stage clinical research (Ashcroft and Pfeffer, 2001).

As the local agencies of one arena of medical self-regulation, RECs operate within a characteristically idiosyncratic web of professional guidance which they may choose to acknowledge or ignore in the pursuit of their appointed task. In terms of standard setting and advice on procedures, the Royal Colleges offer copious assistance. As the originator and promoter of ethics committees, the Royal College of Physicians provides a comprehensive, 80-page set of guidelines (now in its third edition) dealing with, for example, ethical principles, terms of reference, membership, method of working, special classes of research and the use of medical records (Royal College of Physicians, 1996). Other Colleges do the same: the Royal College of Psychiatrists, for example, offering a slim 50-page document with a range of similar advice (Royal College of Psychiatrists, 2000; see also Royal College of Obstetricians and Gynaecologists, 2000b). Most recently, the GMC, in keeping with its statutory responsibility for the standards of medical practice and its ambition to act as the coordinator of medicine's diverse system of governance, has issued its *Research: the role and responsibilities of doctors* with appropriate cross-referencing to other guidance from the profession (General Medical Council, 2002b).

As is customary in the medical profession, the evolution of governance has followed the institutional grain of the existing power structures in ways which suit their *modus operandi* rather than in ways which suit the governance problem to be addressed. So although the regulatory function of standard setting has been much addressed in the research arena, what have been neglected by the profession are the functions of monitoring and intervention (Table 1.1). As we have seen, RECs may or may not decide that the monitoring of projects is part of their remit and that monitoring may or may not be effective (see also Kent, 1997; Pickworth, 2000; Smith *et al.*, 1997). And in terms of intervention, ultimately that responsibility resides with the GMC through its enforcement of sanctions for serious professional misconduct. It is scarcely a seamless process and has provoked considerable internal debate as research governance issues have surfaced.

In 1997, the editors of the *British Medical Journal*, the *Lancet* and *Gut* established the Committee on Publication Ethics (COPE) in response to what they saw as an 'endemic' problem of research fraud in terms of falsification, fabrication and plagiarism (Jones, 1999). Having investigated 56 cases of possible research misconduct, in 1999 COPE produced its guidelines intended to promote and safeguard intellectual honesty at all stages in the research and publication cycle from initial study design onwards (Committee on Publication Ethics, 1999). However, although the issue was thus in the public arena, the debate about who should do what was less easy to resolve. Objectively it could be stated, as did one American observer whilst reflecting on the British experience, that 'the credibility of the [regulatory] process is greatly enhanced by having universally applicable rules, developed and supported by prestigious scientific and medical bodies' and backed by a 'central body which must have the power to review cases and to sanction institutions that do not comply' (Rennie, 1998), but arguments for a national body for research misconduct offended the diversified spirit of medical self-regulation (Smith, 1998). The MRC for one, was swift to point out that it had already devised a specific policy and procedure for handling allegations of scientific misconduct (Evans, 1998; see also Medical Research Council, 1997).

With the revelations about the conduct of medical research produced by the investigations at Bristol Royal Infirmary and Alder Hey, the profession's internal debate was rapidly overtaken by events (see Chapter 6). On 1 March 2001, the Health Minister Philip Hunt announced the publication of the *Research governance framework for health and social care*. Within this framework, RECs are accorded a designated role yet, it is interesting to note, in order to ensure their impartiality remain 'managerially independent of NHS Trust R and D structures' (Department of Health, 2001b: para. 3.12.4). Their work is now overseen by the Central Office for Research Ethics Committees (COREC) working on behalf of the Department of Health to coordinate the development of operational systems for RECs in the NHS in England, manage MRECs, act as a resource for training for REC members and administrators, and provide advice on policy and operational matters relating to RECs (Central Office for Research Ethics Committees, 2002). In July 2001, COREC issued its *Governance arrangements for NHS Research Ethics Committees*, superseding all previous guidance, with the aim of establishing standards and operating procedures that as Sir John Pattison, Director of NHS Research and Development, stated 'are consistent across the UK' (Department of Health, 2000d; Central Office for Research Ethics Committees, 2001). Given the historic variety of RECs, the wealth of guidance from medicine's own regulatory bodies, the problem of which advice to follow first and the natural inertia of what remains an arena of voluntary self-regulation this is clearly one of those ambitions which may remain more in the realm of rhetoric than reality.

Education

Control of the education function, the transmission of medical knowledge, enables the profession to determine what is taught to whom, where, when and how. As a result of these self-regulatory powers, medicine is able, at best, to shape its image and being in ways which suit itself and, at worst, to prevent the state and society from reshaping that identity in ways which the profession itself finds unpalatable. When measured in terms of the sheer quantity of institutions, roles, procedures and networks involved, education is the most complex and impenetrable of the three regulatory arenas. It is unravelled here in terms of workforce planning, undergraduate education and postgraduate education.

Workforce planning

In managerial terms, workforce planning is the means by which the supply of skills is matched to the demand for a service. The medical profession, as is frequently the case, takes a different view and regards workforce planning as the means by which the supply of doctors is matched to the needs of the profession. This fundamental difference reverberates through much of the recent policy debate in this arena.

However, for many years there was little debate simply because the medical, rather than the managerial, definition of workforce planning (or manpower planning as it was then known) prevailed as a natural part of the medical hegemony in policy circles. It was taken as axiomatic that discussion of the medical workforce meant discussion of the medical career structure. And until recently, the medical career structure meant the route by which a doctor achieved full professional recognition as a consultant. Other classes of medical employment were regarded either as stations on the road to that destination or, in the case of GPs, as part of a separate, and lower, professional order. From medicine's perspective, therefore, the hospital career hierarchy was (and to a large degree still is) essentially a training hierarchy and should be planned and organised accordingly. Hence we find that reports on the medical workforce in the NHS focus on the relationship between junior doctor- and consultant-numbers and recommend either restricting the former, or expanding the latter, or both in order to produce a balanced supply of future consultants (see e.g. Department of Health and Social Security, 1987). In general the unchallenged principle was 'that doctors should not be unduly delayed in their progression through the training system' (Department of Health and Social Security, 1987: 87). Only the Short Report of 1981 on medical education took the unusual view that the fundamental issue should be the quality of patient care, not the careers of doctors.

Given the profession's control of the planning bodies themselves this medical view of the workforce world is unsurprising. Although the organisational acronyms may have changed over time, the reality of medical power has not. Beginning in 1984, the central planning function was carried out by the Joint Planning Advisory Committee (JPAC) which had 24 members, 20 of whom were doctors. Until the abolition of RHAs in 1995, the results of JPAC's deliberations were implemented through the Regional Manpower Committees (RMCs), each of which had 11 members and all of whom were doctors (Department of Health and Social Security, 1987: 89). Although JPAC's star subsequently faded and caused it to be replaced by an organisationally impenetrable combination of the Advisory Group on Medical Education, Training and Staffing (AGMETS), the Medical Manpower Standing Advisory Committee (MMSAC) and the Specialist Workforce Advisory Group (SWAG), medical appointments continued to dominate this twilight world between medicine and the state. Indeed, it is perhaps characteristic of medicine's cultural penchant for shadowy complexity as a means for the preservation of its influence that new acronyms continue to appear regularly.

However, despite the profession's comprehensive ring-fencing of the workforce planning activity, the outcome was not an efficient vehicle for medical training to consultant level. Although formally excluded from the planning process, service needs nonetheless exercised an informal influence on the structure of the medical workforce. The service demand for medical pairs of hands has always resulted in more Senior House Officer (SHO) posts than are strictly needed for training purposes and SHOs and registrars have frequently become 'stuck', as it is known, at some point along the long road to consultant status, effectively providing what the Royal College of Surgeons among others has called 'a sub-consultant service' (Royal College of Surgeons of England, 1988: 5). At the same time associate specialist and staff grade appointments have acted as tactfully disguised support for this sub-consultant service. With the advent of the internal market policy and the purchaser–provider divide in 1991, the expression of the service demand on hospitals and the consequent collision with the training demand was formalised through the contract-based purchasing by health authorities of particular services from hospital providers (Figure 5.1). As we shall see in more detail shortly, what the collision clearly demonstrated was that the implementation of the workforce planning function was inextricably intertwined with the operational details of medical training itself. As usual, medical power appeared indivisible.

The obscurity of the medical world of workforce planning meant that for many years it remained undisturbed in its arcane tranquillity. When eventually explored by missionaries of the state in 2000, its topography provoked a response that was predominantly one of disbelief. The consultation report *Health service of all the talents: developing the NHS workforce* described it as 'baffling to the outsider, dealing in currencies (e.g. National Training Numbers) which do not relate easily to the real world'. The report continued: 'The landscape of medical workforce planning is littered with advisory groups which themselves frequently take advice from other bodies whose accountability for the results of their advice is unclear' (Department of Health, 2000c: para. 4.18). Management, it found, remained very much on the periphery of the medical world:

While the needs of the NHS were the prime drivers in planning the workforce for most clinical groups this was not the case for the medical

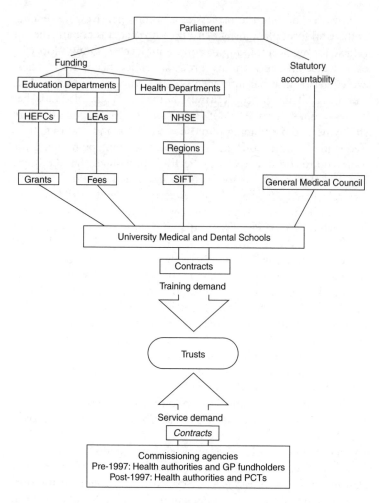

Figure 5.1   Undergraduate medical education

workforce, where the needs of the medical profession were perceived to be dominant. This was reflected in the membership of groups such as AGMETS and SWAG and the weak input from NHS Trusts to medical workforce planning at national level. (Department of Health, 2000c: para. 4.17)

Furthermore, there was a 'lack of proper engagement by many senior NHS managers and policy makers in workforce issues in a way which would be inconceivable in relation, for example, to financial issues' (Department of Health, 2000c: para. 4.16). If proof were needed of what a *Health service of all the talents* called the 'Byzantine' world of medical workforce planning, its model of that world surely provides conclusive evidence (Figure 5.2).

In its attempt to make medical workforce planning part of the NHS planet, the report proposed its integration within a new planning system led by Workforce Development Confederations (WDCs) accountable to a National Workforce Development Board (NWDB) – these were duly established in 2001 (Figure 5.3). The

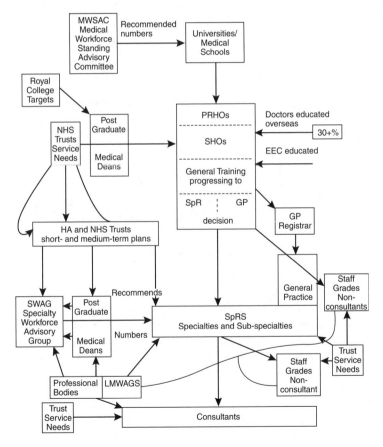

Figure 5.2 Pre-2001 Medical workforce planning arrangements

Source: Department of Health, 2000c.

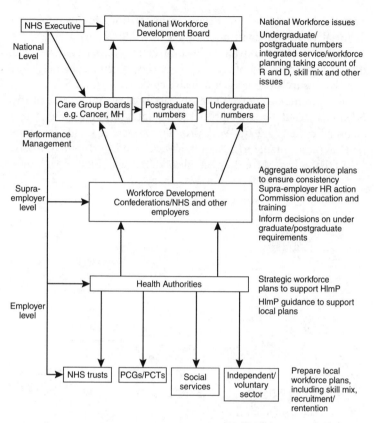

Figure 5.3   Current workforce planning arrangements
Source: Department of Health, 2000c.

NWDB is to determine the number of training commissions required by all professions in the NHS, both medical and non-medical, acting on the advice of the Workforce Numbers Advisory Board (WNAB) which, in turn, is to draw on the plans of the WDCs. Superficially, the invention of these managerial structures gives the impression that the profession has suffered a reduction in its control over its internal composition; one arena of its self-regulatory power has been undermined. However, whether that is indeed the case is doubtful since workforce planning is at present inseparable from the dense power base of medical education and training. It is rather more likely that the new apparatus of workforce planning will sit forlornly alongside the medical structures – parallel and largely impotent.

Both structures are, in any case, being bypassed by the political imperatives of the NHS modernisation programme as it seeks to maximise the political benefits from the large increase in NHS funding announced by Tony Blair in 2000. With little respect for the niceties of workforce planning, *Delivering the NHS plan* set out ambitious plans for net increases by 2008 of 15 000 doctors over the September 2001 baseline (Department of Health, 2002b). This has then been translated into specific targets which the medical training system is asked to deliver. Medical school places are projected to increase by over 43 per cent from 5050 in 1997 to 7250 in 2005 and Specialist Registrar posts by 1000 by 2004 (Review Body on Doctors' and Dentists' Remuneration, 2003: 3, 57). Although the medical profession may not have been party to the construction of these targets, its control of under-graduate and postgraduate education renders it a central player in their realisation.

Undergraduate medical education

Statutory responsibility for the regulation of medical education rests with the Education Committee of the GMC. Section 5 of the Medical Act 1983 states that the Education Committee 'shall have the general function of promoting high standards of medical educa-tion and promoting all stages of medical education' by determining the knowledge and skills, standard of proficiency, and patterns of clinical experience offered by medical schools (Department of Health and Social Security, 1983b, section 5: paras 1 and 2). How-ever, the GMC's ability to regulate this arena is heavily circum-scribed by its need to negotiate with numerous other centres of power involved in the delivery and accreditation of undergraduate education (and even more so, as we shall see, in postgraduate medical education) and which thus control key aspects of the regulatory functions of standard setting, monitoring and intervention: notably, the university medical schools and the Council of Deans of UK Medical Schools and Faculties. Ultimately, the GMC relies heavily on the power of persuasion exercised through 'the issue of Recommendations ... , the convening of conferences and the pro-vision of general advice and encouragement about standards at the national level' (General Medical Council, 1987: 20). Hence its claim that the Education Committee's 'responsibility for standards is linked to provisional and full registration' has to be viewed with caution since in terms of the powers of monitoring and intervention that linkage is decidedly tenuous.

Over time, the GMC's guidance has become more specific and more detailed as it has worked to influence the direction of medical training. *Tomorrow's doctors*, published in 1993, sought to change the emphasis in the curriculum away from gaining knowledge and towards a learning process that includes the ability to evaluate data as well as to develop skills to interact with patients and colleagues (General Medical Council, 1993). Undoubtedly influenced by the events at Bristol and Alder Hey, this guidance was then replaced in 2002 by *Tomorrow's doctors, recommendations on undergraduate education*, which put the principles set out in *Good medical practice* at the centre of undergraduate education (General Medical Council, 2002a). As the GMC has thus raised the profile of its standard-setting function, so it has simultaneously brought to the surface the issue of what ability it has to implement that function. In practice, the Committee's powers are limited to a medical school visit and report for, as a *British Medical Journal* editorial observed whilst commenting on the GMC's difficulties in implementing the curriculum reforms, its 'only [other] sanction is like a nuclear deterrent – it can close a medical school, but it is never going to do that' (British Medical Journal, 1994: 361). The issue is rendered more acute by the fact that, in the UK, graduation from a medical school also confers the right to provisional registration with the GMC and access to clinical practice. This is in contrast to the situation in many other countries where there is a requirement that doctors must pass some form of national assessment before being granted a licence to practise medicine. As Sir Graham Catto, then chairman of the Education Committee observed of the latest guidance, 'we are not proposing a national curriculum nor a national qualifying examination'. He continued, not entirely convincingly, 'There may, however, be other ways of ensuring consistency in the final assessment of clinical skills, such as sharing assessment techniques, without resorting to a national examination' (Catto, 2001). If GMC influence is limited in the period up to graduation, it is even more so in the preregistration house-officer year when graduates are the employees of Trusts and funded by the postgraduate dean. At the end of this period, it is the university, usually in the person of the postgraduate dean, which determines whether to support a graduate's request to move from provisional to full registration. What this rather complex arrangement means in practical political terms is that it is the university which forms the link between standard setting and registration, not the GMC.

The Council's regulatory power is further restricted by the absence of any link between its responsibilities for medical education and the flow of student funds into medical schools (Figure 5.1). Given the separate nature of undergraduate funding which moves from the Education Departments through the Higher Education Funding Councils and the Local Education Authorities and to the universities there is no point of connection between the GMC's regulatory activities and any possible financial sanction for medical schools that do not meet its standards. Add to this the fact that medical schools themselves purchase the practical clinical training of their students through contracts with their local hospital Trusts using Special Increment for Teaching (SIFT) monies allocated by the NHS, and yet further distance emerges between the GMC and the student experience. Bureaucratic separation of the primary elements of governance is thus clear and, it would seem, immutable. In accountability terms, therefore, medical undergraduate education is what might be described as a perfectly disintegrated system. That is not to say that such a mode of organisation is politically dysfunctional. The separation of regulatory functions and powers renders a coordinated state attack on medicine's control of undergraduate education logistically complex, risky and therefore undesirable.

Postgraduate medical education

Postgraduate medical education is quite different. Although the GMC retains responsibility for the Specialist Register (the list of specialist doctors qualified to practise as consultants), all other aspects of postgraduate medical education are part of a fiefdom administered jointly by the medical Royal Colleges and the postgraduate deans using an interlinked system of accreditation, management and financial powers. As with undergraduate education, all roads of accountability lead ultimately to the GMC but, unlike Rome, this does not amount to a statement of GMC power. In its maintenance of the Specialist Register, the GMC is one of four 'competent authorities' constituting the statutory framework for postgraduate medical and dental education, the others being the Specialist Training Authority (STA), the Joint Committee on Postgraduate Training for General Practitioners (JCPTGP) and the General Dental Council (GDC). Established by the European Specialist Medical Qualifications Order 1995, the STA is the UK competent authority for the purposes of specialist medical training and the issue of Certificates of Completion of Specialist Training (CCST) under the terms of the European Medical Directive 93/16EEC. Although the CCST is awarded by the STA as the qualification signifying specialist competence and the right to be admitted to the Specialist Register of the GMC, this accreditation function is dependent on the recommendation of the appropriate Medical Royal College. As one would expect, the Royal Colleges agreed to the establishment of the STA on condition that they lost none of their control over their area of specialist knowledge. At the same time, it is entry on the GMC's Specialist Register (*not* the award of the CCST) that makes the doctor eligible to be appointed to an NHS consultant post, subject to the statutory appointment procedures. So market entry, another significant power to match that of accreditation, is controlled by the GMC. Given this functional complementarity between Royal Colleges and GMC, it follows that the committee structure and membership of the STA should, and does, reflect a balance of power between these two elite groups.

At present, though this will change shortly, general practitioners remain outside this system, there is no GMC register of qualified GPs and, as the state has observed, 'there is little congruity in the arrangements for postgraduate training for general practice and postgraduate training for hospital specialties' (Department of Health, 2001g: para. 20). GPs' training is overseen by the JCPTGP which, on a satisfactory completion of training, issues a general practice Vocational Training Certificate of Prescribed Experience (a VT certificate). As with the STA, the JCPTGP is an independent body, exercising the statutory function of a competent authority on behalf of the state, yet comprised of a balance of medical interests: in this case, the RCGP and the General Practitioners Committee (GPC) of the BMA.

In implementing their responsibilities, the STA and JCPTGP are dependent on an exclusively medical network of organisations and roles which to the managerial mind of *A Health Service of all the talents* is obscurely 'Byzantine' but the 'Green Guide' to postgraduate medical education assembled by the Conference of Postgraduate Medical Deans of the UK (COPMED) and the Academy of Medical Royal Colleges is comprehensible, if complicated (Department of Health, 2000c: para. 4.18; Conference of Postgraduate Medical Deans of the UK, 2002). Negotiated over the past century and a half, these networks are a tribute to the profession's style of regulation by consensus and the accommodation of diverse medical interests in the course of any proffered change.

The educational powers of the 13 Medical Royal Colleges are implemented through an elaborate system of college committees for higher specialist training. In the case of the Royal Colleges of Physicians of Edinburgh and London and the Royal College of Physicians and Surgeons of Glasgow, the operational work is carried out by medical Specialist Advisory Committees (SACs) coordinated by the Joint Committee for Higher Medical Training (JCHMT). A similar arrangement exists for the Royal Colleges of Surgeons of Edinburgh and of England, here coordinated by the Joint Committee on Higher Surgical Training (JCHST). Other Royal Colleges use variations on this organisational theme based on College specialty training committees. The important political point is that the primary unit of epistemic power is the specialty around which other structures are obliged to congregate. This power is reflected in the educational responsibilities of the SACs and other specialist training committees which include the curriculum for training in their specialty; inspection of higher specialist training placements, posts and programmes; recognition and approval of trainers; and recommendations via their College for the award of a CCST (Conference of Postgraduate Medical Deans, 2002: para. 2.7).

At the regional level, the engagement between the work of the SACs and the responsibilities of the postgraduate dean is a vivid illustration of how the world of medicine meets the world of the NHS on medicine's terms. Postgraduate deans are employed jointly by the NHS and universities and are managerially accountable to the Departments of Health for the delivery of postgraduate medical education in the NHS and academically accountable to their respective universities. From a long list, their tasks include: management of the size and distribution of the junior doctor workforce regionally, and nationally through 'Lead Dean' roles related to particular specialties; management of recruitment and appointment to specialist registrar programmes using the entry criteria set by Colleges and Faculties on behalf of the STA; and issuing of the National Training Numbers (NTNs) (and therefore financial support) attached to approved posts. Most importantly, their responsibilities are backed by the power of the state purse. Educational contracts between postgraduate deans and hospital trusts cover 50 per cent of the basic salary of SHOs, SpRs and General Practitioner Registrars (GPRs) and 100 per cent of the salary of Pre-Registration House Officers (PRHOs) as well as funding for postgraduate centres and their staff, libraries and expenses relating to study leave (Paice and Goldberg, 1998).

The harnessing of state financial muscle to the medical interest is achieved through the deanery Specialty Training Committees (STCs) which 'advise' the postgraduate dean on all the key aspects of specialist training such as recruitment, selection, approval and assessment. It would be unwise for any postgraduate dean to act against the advice of their STCs since this would automatically incur the opprobrium of the relevant SAC and College. STC membership is drawn from the specialty concerned (one STC for each specialty as identified by CCST) and includes College regional or specialty advisers and representatives of the relevant SACs – ensuring, as COPMeD innocently puts it, 'a useful fusion of values and roles' (Conference of Postgraduate Medical Deans of the UK, 2002: para. 3). Whilst, at deanery level, College regional and specialty advisers facilitate the integration of the profession's self-regulatory structures with the resources of the state, within hospital Trusts that integration is achieved through the relationship between College tutors (appointed by and accountable to particular Colleges) and the postgraduate dean's clinical tutor (a consultant who is both an employee of the Trust and accountable to the dean for the delivery of the Trust's educational contract). In addition, many Colleges insist that a consultant who acts as clinical supervisor for a trainee has acquired College approval for the performance of that role.

GP training is organised somewhat differently from specialist training but the principles of professional control and subordination of the state interest are common to both areas. Directors of Postgraduate General Practice Education are accountable to the postgraduate deans and are responsible for organising and monitoring GP training. They act on the advice of the General Practice Education Committees which recommend posts for general practice training drawing on information from the JCPTGP. At the local level, GP course organisers and GP tutors coordinate and provide the training activity. Unlike the other Medical Royal Colleges, the RCGP does not have a direct curriculum planning and accreditation role. Working through and with the JCPTGP, its indirect influence is nonetheless considerable.

Although comprehensively integrated with the managerial apparatus of the postgraduate dean, the Medical Royal Colleges are not, however, dependent on that machinery for the exercise of their educational power. Independently of the dean, Colleges determine which junior doctor posts in hospital Trusts are 'approved' for training, and which not. Each approved post carries an accreditable value – the period of accreditable higher specialist training that can be gained in each specialty for which the post is approved – and the withdrawal of College approval means that, for training purposes, the post ceases to exist. The exercise of this sanction in circumstances where a College deems that a post, and the resources attached to it, no longer meets its educational criteria generates much political heat since it is a clear assertion that the medical world can and does make its regulatory decisions independently of service need. In its consultation document *Postgraduate medical education and training* on the proposed reforms of medical education and training, the Department of Health noted that

> educational decisions in setting standards or in judging whether individual training locations, training programmes and individual doctors have met those standards have profound effects on the viability of hospitals and therefore on other local health services – if an Accident and Emergency Unit loses training approval, the hospital is unable to employ any 'training grade' doctors in that Unit and may not be able to deliver important services to a local community. (Department of Health, 2001g: para. 23)

Not surprisingly, in its response to the consultation the medical profession rejected this implied slur on its good name maintaining that 'the current system worked well' and that 'withdrawal [of training accreditation] is not carried out in a peremptory or unnecessary way' (Department of Health, 2001h: para. 12).

Medicine's dominance of the operational details of specialist training coupled with its retention of the separate power of training accreditation has meant that change can only occur if the interests of the medical elites (principally the Medical Royal Colleges and the GMC) are an intrinsic part of the proposed reform. As Stacey has observed of educational change in medicine, 'the felt need to consult and consult again in order to reach consensus decisions greatly slows down the decision making process' (Stacey, 1992a: 250–1). Nine years after the Calman report on higher specialist training proposed significant changes to the training of specialist registrars in 1993 (Working Group on Medical Specialist Training, 1993), a second report in 2002 (appropriately entitled *Unfinished business*) recommended that perhaps there should also be reform of SHO training (Department of Health, 2002h). Consultation on these proposals are continuing with the Academy of Medical Royal Colleges (AMRC) acting as facilitator of the political conversation between medicine and state. Meanwhile, and linked with this, the state's bullish statement in *The NHS Plan* that 'We will rationalise the complex arrangements for medical education' by replacing the JCPTGP and STA with the new Medical Education Standards Board has evolved into more conciliatory linguistic form as the necessary engagement with medical power has occurred (Department of Health, 2000b: para. 8.28). In 2003, a 'Memorandum of Understanding' between the Department of Health and the AMRC 'laid the foundations for the good partnership working needed to take forward policy on postgraduate medical education' and the establishment of what is to be called the Postgraduate Medical Education and Training Board (PMETB) (Department of Health, 2003a).

Performance

It is a central tenet of the political bargain between medicine and the state that the profession will regulate, and be seen to regulate, its standards of performance to a level acceptable to civil society so that public trust in doctors is maintained. Should it not do so, then the state will be obliged to intervene to protect the interest of civil society. Much of the recent debate about the medical profession has focused on its regulation of performance: that is, the way in which doctors apply the knowledge they have acquired through research and education. That debate is dealt with in detail in Chapter 6 building on the understanding of the profession's historic approach to performance regulation presented here.

The 1858 Medical Act established the GMC and gave it the right and the duty to determine and regulate medicine's professional standards. Financed by the profession itself and answerable to Parliament through the Privy Council, the GMC controls entry to, and exit from, the profession by maintaining a register of doctors fit to practise medicine. Following successful completion of the pre-registration year, an individual's name is entered on the Register and can be removed only if the GMC's Professional Conduct Committee judges him or her guilty of 'serious professional misconduct' (General Medical Council, 1993). The law requires all doctors to be registered before they may practise.

Until the 1978 Medical Act, all cases of suspected fitness to practise were dealt with by two GMC committees: the Preliminary Proceedings Committee (PPC) which decides if there is a *prima facie* case to answer and the Professional Conduct Committee (PCC) which undertakes a full inquiry into the practitioner's continued fitness to practice. Since the 1978 Act, where the alleged unfitness is thought to be caused by ill health (physical or mental, including alcohol and drug addiction), the case is dealt with by the Health Committee, adding an extra dimension to the regulation of performance. Nonetheless, the limitation of these procedures was that they excluded continued poor performance by a doctor who was not sick. Historically, the GMC had always been slow to examine the clinical aspects of complaints and reluctant to accept that serious incompetence amounted to serious professional misconduct (Stacey, 2000: 34).

From 1983 onwards when Nigel Spearing MP began a campaign for a lesser charge than serious professional misconduct to be included in the Council's fitness to practise procedures, the GMC came under regular pressure to introduce reform as the media found new scandals and exposures (Stacey, 1992a: 182–3). However, as with other aspects of the regulation of medicine, change was slow in forthcoming. In part this was because it was not until 1993 that the state felt sufficiently energised to add its own voice to the demands for reform, and even then this was fairly muted. In that year, problems with South Birmingham's pathology service caused the Secretary of State for Health to request a review by the Department's Chief Medical Officer (CMO) of guidance in relation to the identification of poor performance of doctors (CMO's Review Group, 1995: 7). Given that the majority of the Review Group were leading members of medicine's elites, its subsequent report *Maintaining medical excellence* can be viewed as a clear recognition by the profession that the pressures from the state were real and required a tangible response.

Twelve years after Nigel Spearing launched his campaign, the 1995 Medical (Professional Performance) Act gave the GMC the powers to introduce the Performance Review Procedure designed to enhance its ability to detect and correct inappropriate standards in the delivery of clinical care by doctors (GMC, 1997a,b; see also Stacey, 1992b). The new procedure allows for a range of corrective actions to be taken once the nature of a doctor's poor performance had been established, ranging from retraining to, eventually, removal from the register. On the other hand, its potential scope, and hence its political utility, is limited by its focus not just on poor performance, but on 'seriously deficient performance'.

This increase in the range of behaviours for which doctors' self-regulation holds them formally accountable has been paralleled by a significant, and GMC-sponsored, revision of the role of the medical peer group in that process of accountability. Up to the early 1980s, members of the medical profession were advised by the GMC not to report each other in the name of professional unity (Stacey, 2000: 34). Critics of this ruling, notably an outspoken member of the GMC, Mrs Jean Robinson, argued that this led to a culture of 'secrecy and deceit' and encouraged the non-reporting of serious cases of malpractice (Robinson, 1999). After 1983 the advice was modified and, eventually, completely reversed in 1995 in *Good medical practice* where the duties and responsibilities of doctors are codified (General Medical Council, 1995). This makes quite clear that a practitioner who has evidence that another is incompetent to practise for whatever reason, or is not practising ethically, has a responsibility to take action. Doctors are advised that: 'You must protect patients when you believe that a colleague's conduct, performance or health is a threat to them'.

Further detailed guidance then follows, concluding, 'The safety of patients must come first at all times' (General Medical Council, 1995: paras 18, 19). The interest of patients is thus formally placed before the interest of medical colleagues and the role of the peer group becomes one of patient protection rather than doctor protection – an important cultural shift.

In the pre-Bristol era, the GMC's ability to translate external demands for change in the regulation of doctors' poor performance into lengthy internal wrangles resulted in a leisurely approach to the business of reform. It was aided in the perpetuation of this style by the subordination of the NHS's own disciplinary procedures to those of the medical world, the dominance of NHS procedures by doctors and hence the absence of any substantial alternative to the self-regulatory option.

The NHS has three categories of disciplinary procedures dealing with doctors' performance: personal misconduct, professional misconduct and professional incompetence. Personal misconduct, such as assault or sexual harassment, falls within the remit of the employer's internal disciplinary procedures. Professional misconduct or incompetence involving the exercise of clinical skills, however, are accorded a separate disciplinary status to that of other NHS employees and are dealt with by a complex set of procedures contained in two government circulars (Department of Health and Social Security, 1982; Department of Health, 1990b). The procedures invoked under the guidance of these circulars are either, in the less serious cases, a form of medical peer review or, where they could result in dismissal, are in the words of the only formal study of this issue: 'legalistic, time consuming, expensive, and intimidating to those who might wish to report a problem or who might have something relevant to say on the matter' (Donaldson, 1994a: 1281). Further problems in implementing the procedures arise from the difficulty of establishing a clinician's performance, the automatic closing of ranks by a doctor's peers and, in the case of sick doctors, reluctance on the part of doctors to activate a procedure with disciplinary connotations (Donaldson, 1994a: 1280, 1994b).

Although notionally management led, the NHS's disciplinary procedures have in practice been dominated by doctors (Allsop and Mulcahy, 1996: 107–12). It was, therefore, perfectly normal for the GMC's introduction of its new performance procedures in July 1997 to be followed by Departmental guidance to the chief executives of provider Trusts in December 1997 on how they could best facilitate the implementation of the profession's policy (NHSE, 1997). In a sympathetic bureaucratic dance, the NHSE's guidance to the NHS exactly mirrored that of the GMC's guidance to Health Authorities and Trusts (General Medical Council, 1997b). There could be no doubt as to who was the lead partner. Managers were assumed to be at worst passive and at best helpful in the business of self-regulation. Indeed, there was no reason why managers should think otherwise given the NHSE's formal respect for clinical autonomy. For example, in its statement on clinical guidelines, theoretically a possible means for performance monitoring, the NHSE is at pains to emphasise its respect for doctors' control of their own labour space:

> clinical guidelines can still only assist the practitioner; they cannot be used to mandate, authorise or outlaw treatment options. Regardless of the strength of the evidence, it will remain the responsibility of the practising clinicians to interpret their application ... It would be wholly inappropriate for clinical guidelines to be used as a means of coercion of the individual clinician by managers and senior professionals. (NHSE, 1996: 10)

Historically, the Medical Royal Colleges and GMC had long accepted a tacit political agreement that whilst the former controlled the regulatory territory of postgraduate education the latter ruled the realm of performance. But even before the events of Bristol and Alder Hey caused a radical reappraisal of this divide, strains were already being felt. It was becoming apparent that if a positive as well as a negative approach to performance was to be taken in the interest of maintaining public trust in doctors, then the regulatory arenas of education and performance would have to develop joint forms of engagement. In particular the Royal Colleges began to argue that prevention is better than cure and that performance monitoring should be aiming at maintaining best practice rather than concentrating solely on those who fall below a given standard.

In this respect, the developing area of CME (part of the Royal Colleges' domain) began to be viewed as a form of intervention capable of dealing with some of the issues prevalent in the performance regulatory arena. In 1994 Kenneth Calman, then

Chief Medical Officer, placed CME at the heart of the triangle of forces between medicine, society and state when he argued that whereas in previous years the legitimacy of a doctor's clinical competence was assured by the very fact of registration, now a 'more formal' and continuous system is required to assuage public doubts:

> The case for CME rests heavily on the concept of confidence: clinicians must command the confidence of the patients they treat; of the public as a whole; of the hospital managers to whom they are accountable for the quality of services to patients; and NHS managers who contract with hospitals on behalf of patients must have confidence in the quality of the service they buy. (Calman, 1994: 6)

But if CME was to be used as a vehicle both for reassuring the public and for expanding the regulatory territory of the Colleges then it would have to be consistent, comprehensive and mandatory, and seen to be so – a tall order for 13 fiercely independent institutions. By the mid-1990s the Colleges had evolved different systems of CME, achieved different levels of compliance among their members and introduced different sanctions for non-compliance with CME regulations. Those sanctions included: exclusion from being considered for merit awards and College committee membership (Royal College of Obstetricians and Gynaecologists), loss of teaching status (Royal College of Opthalmologists) and viewing a consultant without CME accreditation as a reason for the non-approval of training posts with which they are associated (Royal College of Physicians) (Ward, 1994). However, since the logic of any regulatory intervention is that it must, ultimately, be linked to registration, there remained the unresolved issue of how the CME accrediting powers of the Colleges could be linked to the registration power of the GMC. As we shall see in Chapter 6, this issue was to form a key part of the revalidation debate.

Conclusions

Until comparatively recently, medicine's system of self-regulation constituted an invisible world which paralleled, and remained largely aloof from, the political vicissitudes which constantly shake the all too apparent world of the NHS. In principle accountable to

Parliament through the GMC, but in practice for much of its existence accountable only to itself, self-regulation has progressed through numerous phases of evolution characterised not so much by survival of the fittest as by the accommodation of diversity. As a result, it is populated by a rich variety of institutional flora and fauna which coexist in an environment which, until Bristol, Alder Hey and other events cast their long shadow, was equable and supportive.

Since neither time nor efficiency were recognisable imperatives, each of the regulatory species of research, education and perform- ance could evolve at their own pace, reliant on the undemanding principle of consensus to respond to the influences in their partic- ular locale and so order their development and their direction. Quite different identities have emerged. In terms of the normal timescale of medical self-regulatory evolution, research has only just emerged: the first arrangements for its governance were only formalised in the mid-1970s. Unlike education and performance, it did not possess a distinct national agency capable of imposing even the semblance of uniformity on the activities of RECs. Subsequently, both the Colleges and the GMC chose to interpret their responsibilities for standards as including research and there- fore issued professional guidance, but this has not encouraged the development of the complex of institutional roles and procedures so characteristic of the arenas of education and performance and so attractive to the profession's politicians. There is no career opportunity in research regulation.

Not so in the arena of education. Here there are a variety of openings. In terms of the regulation of the number of doctors which should be entering medical education, again a relatively recent (1980s) innovation, national bodies such as JPAC and SWAG required medical practitioners to staff them – though their life expectation tended to be short. From medicine's perspective, it was perfectly natural that workforce planning, as it became known, should serve the needs of medical education and therefore should form part of the medical world. Afterall, both undergradu- ate and postgraduate education took a view on what was needed in terms of training numbers and these readily filtered into the activities of the planning bodies. That these views might not coin- cide with a patient-centred and service-led approach to workforce planning did not register in the policy discourse until *A health service of all the talents* in 2000. Thereafter, the ambitious projections of doctor numbers required to deliver the promises of *The NHS plan* (and so realise the political profit from the expanded investment in the Health Service) imposed a set of targets which, for the time being at least, now drive the business of medical workforce planning.

However, the expansion of the medical workforce is dependent on the cooperation of the structures of undergraduate and postgraduate education that, although both ultimately the responsibility of the Education Committee of the GMC, remain determinedly separate domains of the medical world with quite different regulatory identities. Undergraduate education is firmly ensconced in the province of universities and is subject to only a distant guiding influence from the GMC – an influence further diluted by the separation of the funding power (which derives from the higher education funding councils) from the GMC's statutory validation and registration powers. Its evolution has therefore been shaped far more by the general experience of higher education than by any peculiarly medical culture. However, as one moves from undergraduate to postgraduate education, so one crosses a clear territorial boundary into a province where the historic accreditation powers of the Medical Royal Colleges (largely implemented through the JCHMT, the JCHST and the SACs) and the postgraduate deans' control of NHS training funds have combined to foster a dense self-regulatory jungle. Overlapping roles and structures exist in abundance, confusing and disorientating to any potential intruder. But through them run many paths, visible to the insider, which lead eventually to the CCST and the GMC's Specialist Register.

Whilst the Royal Colleges have dominated the regulatory arena of education, the GMC has retained and enhanced its control of performance. Working within the gradualist tradition of medical reform, it has enlarged its definition of performance (and hence its regulatory territory) to include not just 'serious professional misconduct' but ill health and poor performance as well. Fresh committees and procedures have been grafted on to the Council's body politic and medical interests accommodated as the incremental process of change has moved forward. As the statutory lynchpin of medicine's edifice of governance, the GMC was duty bound to respond to issues of public trust in doctors and this, in its own time, it did.

But as one part of a dispersed system of medical powers the Council could not guarantee that the apparatus of self-regulation as a whole would also recognise the significance of a decline in public support for the profession and therefore the need to re-engineer the relationship between civil society, medicine and the state. One of the political strengths of the world of medicine is the fragmentation of its formal regulatory functions, its reliance on informal professional networks, its multiple loci of power and hence the difficulties inherent in any state ambition to take it over. By the same token, one of the political weaknesses of medicine is the absence of any coordinating body capable of producing a unified response to pressures for reform and managing the politics of change. How, therefore, would it respond to a concerted attack on its power?

6

The invasion of medical territory

Introduction

By 1997 it was clear that the internal market reforms of the Conservative government would not attempt to challenge medical power in the heartland of clinical practice. The logic of the triangular relationship between medicine, civil society and the state had reasserted itself and the state was once again obliged to recognise that the delivery of its promises to its citizens was dependent on the goodwill of the medical profession. Even at the ambitious height of the reforms, no policy had been proposed which would have seriously intruded on the many aspects of medical territory either outside or within the NHS. As a principle, self-regulation remained a sacred tenet of the NHS faith and the quality of clinical practice a matter for medical initiates alone to judge, presided over by their high priests and ordered according to their historic rituals.

The retention of this key element of professional autonomy meant that doctors remained in a strong position to negotiate and maintain their economic autonomy (their market and occupational advantages) and their political autonomy (their influence over policy). At the same time the legal and cultural assumptions which underpinned these autonomies continued to dominate the day-to-day life of the Health Service, regardless of radical political rhetoric and of the superficial tides of the managerial discourse. The worlds of doctors and managers coexisted, with the latter a minor political satellite in the orbit of medical power.

The arrival of a Labour government in May 1997 challenged all that, partly because there has always been a Labour Party scepticism regarding the privileges of doctors but, more importantly, because a policy window of opportunity opened as a result of an unprecedented and sustained media interest in the quality of doctors' work and the mobilisation of the normally quiescent contribution of civil society to the triangle of forces between itself, medicine and the state. Once opened, this particular window allowed the state to initiate a range of policy invasions into the hallowed territory of medical self-regulation. In analysing the path of the ensuing confrontation between medicine and the state, this chapter begins by considering the nature of the political impetus generated by the events at Bristol, Alder Hey and elsewhere and their implications for public trust in the profession. Second, it examines how the state sought to translate that impetus into aggressive regulatory policies but then found itself propelled by forces it could not control. Third, the chapter deals with medicine's initial, divided response to this situation and then, finally, with the profession's coalescence around its own policy of revalidation and the consequent and undignified retreat of the state from medical territory.

The policy window opens

Traditionally, the regulation by medicine of its own affairs had never been an item likely to get on to the policy agenda. As one of the key assumptions of the 1948 concordat between medicine and state, clinical autonomy and all that flowed from it had been a constant among the vicissitudes of the post-Griffiths era. *Working for patients*, the White Paper which initiated the 1991 reforms, made no attempt to challenge the principle of self-regulation but emphasised that 'the quality of medical work should be reviewed by a doctor's peers' (Department of Health, 1989a: 40). Throughout the early and mid-1990s, medicine's autonomous system of professional governance continued on its serene course, largely unhindered by the storms afflicting the NHS's formal accountability structures. Nonetheless, the state's acceptance of what had always been was tinged by an awareness that self-regulation itself might require reform (see Chapter 5).

At this point, the state's attitude did not evoke any sense of great urgency: change was necessary but did not demand drastic measures. However, the election of the 1997 Labour government immediately altered the style of the political proceedings.

The 1997 White Paper *The new NHS: modern, dependable* stated that the government would seek 'to strengthen the existing systems of professional self-regulation by ensuring that they are *open, responsive and publicly accountable*' (Department of Health, 1997a: 59, emphasis added). It was therefore clear from the outset that the state under Labour wanted to curb the professional independence of doctors. The reform of medical self-regulation was, it appeared, now very much on the state's health care policy agenda. But then, it could be said, so was a lot else.

The translation of professional autonomy from one item on a crowded policy agenda to a priority issue that would drive a raft of other policy initiatives occurred not because of the state's aspirations but because of a sustained engagement between the media, doctors' performance and civil society which then impacted on the policy process. The Labour government may have been preparing for an invasion of medical territory but in the event its hand was forced.

On 29 May 1998, the GMC ruled that two surgeons from Bristol Royal Infirmary were guilty of continuing to operate on children with heart defects when they knew their death rates were unacceptably high. In addition, a doctor manager was found guilty of failing to stop the operations after he had been alerted to the high mortality. Accompanied by intense media interest, these decisions sent what the *British Medical Journal* described as 'nothing short of an earthquake through British medicine' commenting with some foresight that 'the reverberations are likely to be felt for years' (British Medical Journal, 1998a). Public trust in doctors would, it seemed, never be the same again. All had changed, 'changed utterly' (British Medical Journal, 1998b: 1917). In the following month, faced with an unprecedented degree of public concern over the issue, the government announced that a formal inquiry, armed with a wide-ranging brief and considerable investigative resources, would be conducted into the management of complex paediatric heart surgery at the Bristol Royal Infirmary Trust and its predecessor between 1984 and 1995. The policy window had opened. Other events were to ensure that it did not close.

To the media, the attractions of the Bristol Inquiry were many. It was lavishly resourced (£14 million over three years), there was no easy answer to the questions it posed, its subject was children and therefore emotive, its chair was Sir Ian Kennedy (not a close friend of the medical profession), it was surrounded by local parental action groups, and, above all, it could be linked to other 'dangerous doctor' stories – of which there were now a plentiful supply. Amid the plethora of cases of inadequate medical performance illuminated by legal action, GMC investigations, local Trust inquiries and independent inquiries in the period following the Bristol revelations, two stand out as having particular significance for public trust in the profession: the Royal Liverpool Children's Hospital Trust, Alder Hey and the GP, Dr Harold Shipman.

In September 1999, following the early findings of the Bristol Inquiry that parents had not given their properly informed consent for the hospital's retention of their children's organs, parents of children treated at Alder Hey Hospital initiated a series of actions which resulted, first, in a CMO investigation into the national situation regarding the retention of organs, body parts and tissues at post-mortem examinations and, second, in an inquiry chaired by Mr Michael Redfern QC into what had happened at Alder Hey itself (Royal Liverpool Children's Hospital Inquiry, 2001). The Redfern Inquiry revealed that between 1988 and 1995 the pathologist at Alder Hey, Professor van Velzen, had removed the hearts, brains and other internal organs from all the 850 children on whom he had conducted a post-mortem, ostensibly for research purposes, without the consent of their parents. As we have seen in Chapter 3, local patient lobby groups provided the media with ample means with which to maintain the political visibility of the issue (see Chapter 3). But its significance lies not only in its contribution to the pressure for policy change, but also in what it tells us about the changing relationship between civil society and medicine. In other words, it provides important insights into why the triangle of forces has become destabilised and why a policy response was thus required. For behind the issue of organ retention is a collision between the established practice and culture of the medical profession as enshrined in dimly perceived laws and the emergent expectations of citizens founded on new conceptions of health care rights and the ownership of the body.

In 2000, the CMO's national census of organs and tissues held by pathology services in England revealed the retention for research and teaching purposes of approximately 105 000 organs, body parts, stillbirths and fetuses of which the relatives concerned were largely unaware (Chief Medical Officer, 2001: 22).

The experience of parents at Bristol and Alder Hey was therefore not unique: it was established medical practice for children (and adults) to be interred having had their organs removed but with the relatives believing they had been buried intact. Propelled by the media, what the Bristol and Alder Hey Inquiries did was to transfer this customary activity from the private medical sphere to the public sphere where the high profile politicisation of pathology duly took place. As politicisation occurred, it threw into sharp relief the political role of the law in sustaining a particular definition of the patient–doctor relationship.

Hospital post-mortems were, and are, legally governed by the Human Tissues Act 1961 (though in practice post-mortems are subject to interim guidance from the Department of Health hastily issued in March 2000). For the purposes of this Act, the active consent of relatives for a post-mortem examination to take place is not needed; it must simply be established that the relatives do not object to such an examination. There is no express requirement to give particular information to the relatives nor is there a legal limit to the amount of 'tissue' that can be retained. Legally, the person who is, in the words of the Act, 'in possession of the body' can be the hospital rather than the relatives and a member of the hospital staff can therefore authorise the removal of organs and tissues (Chief Medical Officer, 2001: 10).

The law in this field therefore reflects and supports the permissive and pervasive nature of traditional medical authority. It may be, as the CMO's report stimulated by the Bristol and Alder Hey events observed, that 'the law in this area is old-fashioned, ambiguous and tilted towards marginalising families rather than ensuring that they are equal partners in the decision making process' (Chief Medical Officer, 2001: 6). But, equally, it can be said that pre-Bristol the law was very much in line with medical culture. Commenting on the Pathology Department at Bristol Royal Infirmary and its continued involvement in the removal and retention of human material without the real awareness of parents, the interim report of the Bristol Inquiry stated:

> We may regret that those standards were the product of a small group of professionals talking to themselves. We may agree that they reflected a degree of professional arrogance. We may lament that they displayed a lack of interest in, or paternalism towards, the views and

feelings of parents. *But that was how things were. That was the culture of the times.* (Bristol Royal Infirmary Inquiry, 2000: 56, emphasis added)

As the intensity of the exchanges between the Bristol and Alder Hey lobby groups and NHS management indicate, this was not a culture shared by many of the parents involved. For health consumers such as these, consent really did mean 'informed consent' and not the 'lack of objection' definition enshrined in the Human Tissue Act 1961. As Professor Ian Booth of the Royal College of Paediatrics and Child Health reflected, the implication for the medical profession was clear:

> From our perspective there has been a very large change in the extent to which the public wish to be informed and consulted, or perhaps it is a change in their ability to voice that need which has probably always been there, and we support that very much. We would accept that in many cases the profession has been slow to keep up with that big cultural change. (Chief Medical Officer, 2001: 27)

In his House of Commons statement in January 2001 on the publication of the Alder Hey Inquiry report, the Secretary of State for Health, Alan Milburn, noted that 'The NHS can no longer assume that the benefits of science, medicine or research are somehow self-evident regardless of the wishes of parents or their families. The relationship between patients and the service today has to be based on informed consent' (Secretary of State for Health, 2001). Medical values, it can be said, were no longer absolute but contingent upon those of the health consumer.

Cultural dissonance between patients and doctors was now a force for policy change and public trust in the medical profession, a key political issue. So much so that for the politicians it was no longer a question of their taking advantage of a policy window on the reform of medical self-regulation but rather one of attempting to restrict the size of the window for which they would be held to account. They were in danger of losing control of a political dynamic with its own inbuilt momentum. The policy agenda was large and growing. In his same Commons statement responding to Alder Hey, Milburn noted that the clash between modern patient expectations and traditional clinical practice 'will require changes in practice and changes in policy. It will require changes in medical education ... it will also require changes to the law' (Secretary of State for Health, 2001).

Amid the almost daily reportings of doctors failing their patients at this time, one other event in particular acted to sustain the political pressure for reform. On 31 January 2000 Dr Harold Shipman, a general practitioner, received 15 life sentences for murdering 15 of his middle-aged and elderly women patients by lethal injections of diamorphine. Subsequently the first report by the Shipman Inquiry established that the GP had in fact killed 215 of his patients (Shipman Inquiry, 2002a). Although to the detached observer it may be apparent that murderers make up their own rules to create the space required, nonetheless the Shipman trial reinforced the impression in the public mind that when it came to the control and disposal of the human body at and after the point of death, doctors enjoyed a distinct social advantage. Shipman was able illicitly to stockpile large quantities of controlled drugs, kill his patients, avoid a referral to a coroner for a post-mortem in all but a very few cases, and arrange the cremation of his victims in the majority of cases, all undetected. Dame Janet Smith, the chair of the Shipman Inquiry, commented: 'As a general practitioner, Shipman was trusted implicitly by his patients and their families. He betrayed their trust in a way and to an extent that I believe is unparalleled in history' (Shipman Inquiry, 2002a: para. 14.21). As with Bristol and Alder Hey, the Shipman case illustrated with brutal clarity the large areas of discretion afforded to doctors by the public's trust in them as self-governing professionals. Moreover it is, as the Inquiry has demonstrated, a discretion woven in the fabric of the procedures for death and cremation certification which assume and are dependent upon the integrity of the medical professional using them (Shipman Inquiry, 2002b).

What the Bristol, Alder Hey and Shipman Inquiries also illustrated was the size and complexity of any putative external intervention into the self-governing territory of medicine, particularly if that intervention was undertaken without the consent and cooperation of the inhabitants. As Chapter 5 has described, the system of medical self-regulation is characterised both by its own institutions, values and rules and by a mirror image of legal, cultural and procedural freedoms within the structure of the NHS. Despite the coincidence of state aspirations and civil society discontent, the construction of a policy response to the demonstrable limitations of self-regulation was always going to be an exercise for which there was no historical precedent and no certain political pathway.

The state's policy response

Not surprisingly, therefore, the initial policy response followed the well-trodden path of proposing bureaucratic controls which would operate through the normal line-management system of the NHS, the radical difference being that they would deal with clinical standards rather than finance, the normal focus of the accountability system. Thus in April 1998 it was announced that 'for the first time in the history of the NHS' hospital Trusts were to be held legally accountable for the quality of the service they provided (Department of Health, 1998a). (The requirement was subsequently given statutory force by the Health Act, 1999.) In the consultation document *A first class service: quality in the new NHS* which followed this announcement it was made clear that what was proposed was a management-led system of clinical governance designed to set and monitor clinical standards (Department of Health, 1998b). Its definition of the new managerial concept of clinical governance was of 'a framework through which NHS organisations are accountable for continuously improving the quality of their services and safeguarding high standards of care by creating an environment in which excellence in clinical care will flourish' (Department of Health, 1998b: 33). Self-regulation remained, at least in name, but the document notes that if the public confidence in doctors so seriously dented by events such as those at Bristol is to be restored, self-regulation must be modernised. It must be situated within a state-administered apparatus of accountability to ensure that it is 'open to public scrutiny; responsive to changing clinical practice and changing service needs; and publicly accountable for professional standards set nationally and the action taken to maintain those standards' (Department of Health, 1998b: para. 3.44). Furthermore, if necessary (and, one assumes, should the profession prove uncooperative), clinical governance 'will provide a systematic framework that can be extended into the clinical community at all levels' (Department of Health, 1998b: para. 3.12).

Perhaps the bravest statement in this opening policy formation salvo was that 'Government will take responsibility for clarifying which treatments work best' (Department of Health, 1998b: para. 2.27). By proposing to take ultimate responsibility for clinical standards, a key area in the control of medical knowledge, the state was making crystal clear its ambition to redefine the contract between medicine and the state and gain sovereignty over some or all of medicine's self-governing knowledge territory. What the state had not grasped at this stage was the extent and complexity of that territory. As Table 1.1 summarises, and Chapter 5 has elaborated, the territory contains the application of the governance functions of standard setting, monitoring and intervention to the knowledge arenas of research, education and performance. Control of this territory in turn provides the basis for medicine's negotiation and maintenance of its economic and, to an extent, its political autonomy (see Chapter 1). Invasion of the medical domain was therefore going to require detailed planning and coordinated logistical support. Policy implementation would be a demanding business.

As the policy technicians began to work out how the policy of clinical governance might be implemented, and thus a realistic challenge to medical hegemony mounted, the extent of its complexities began to emerge. An initial problem was that the actual process of clinical governance was not defined in the early policy statements which had focused instead on its intended output of enhanced service quality. Thus, clinical governance was at various times taken to include medical audit, clinical audit, critical incident reporting, adverse event reporting, risk management, annual appraisal and quality assurance – in other words, anything which could be understood to maintain and improve clinical standards. Structures and theoretical responsibilities were easier for the policy technicians to deal with and can be summarised here in terms of their intended governance functions. In somewhat cavalier style, responsibilities for these functions were allocated as follows: for standard setting, to the National Institute for Clinical Excellence (NICE) and the National Service Frameworks (NSFs); for monitoring and evaluation, to the Health Authorities (HAs), PCGs, the NHSE, CHI, the NHS Performance Assessment Framework and the National Patient and User Survey; and for intervention, to the previous list for evaluation plus the provider hospital and

PCTs themselves (National Health Service Executive, 1999a: 4, 1999b: 3). Regrettably, no one knew how these different structures and their overlapping functions were intended to interrelate. There was no coordinating system of accountability.

Part of the political problem was that the early development of the clinical governance policy was overtaken by the tide of events which had begun with the GMC decision on the Bristol consultants. As one dangerous doctor story followed another, the state was forced into policy formation on the hoof. It did not have the political space and time to plan its invasion of medical territory properly, it had underestimated what was involved and the initial tactic of scapegoating the medical profession, particularly the GMC, had a finite half-life as a means for dealing with public pressure. At the same time, the aggressive intent of forcing medicine's system of self-regulation to integrate with the as yet unknown arrangements for NHS clinical governance had, with the exception of the GMC, produced a predictably unenthusiastic response from medicine's elites who, as we shall see shortly, had their own internal divisions to address. The policy window may have opened, but it had left the state, as much as medicine, exposed to the chill winds of citizen disapproval.

The Department's *Supporting doctors, protecting patients*, a consultation paper produced in November 1999, shows in graphic detail the extent of the state's exposure at this time. In blissful ignorance of what was to come the document cites two cases which 'can be regarded as a watershed in the history of poor clinical performance in the NHS' (a statement which is in itself a powerful indicator of the formative capacity of particular issues): the Bristol children's heart surgery service and the gynaecologist dismissed by South Kent Hospitals NHS Trust because of serious failures in his clinical practice (Mr Rodney Ledward, the subject of an inquiry chaired by Miss Jean Ritchie QC). As the document admits, the main difficulty in developing an NHS policy, clinical governance or otherwise, to deal with such cases was the absence of any obvious starting point.

> Present NHS procedures for detecting and dealing with poor clinical performance are fragmented and inflexible. There is a strong impression that some doctors who are performing poorly are slipping through the net because employers are not willing to use daunting disciplinary

procedures, because it is difficult to hold the employee to account or because no adequate procedures exist, because other health professionals are reluctant to report a colleague's problems, or because the systems to detect poor performance or underlying ill health are just not adequate. (Department of Health, 1999a: para. 2.55)

And, it can be added, the procedures which do exist are largely controlled by doctors (Allsop and Mulcahy, 1996: chapters 2 and 3). In a sense this is what one would expect. Given that the role of NHS management had never before included the monitoring of clinician performance, since this was understood to be the province of self-regulation, management-driven performance procedures were superfluous to the historic understanding of how the Health Service worked.

Supporting doctors, protecting patients marks the point at which the self-belief of the Labour government in its ability to use management action as the sole means of affecting change in the governance of medicine began to evaporate. (It is significant that the consultation document was produced under the aegis of the CMO who acts as a bridge between state and profession.) As the document's long list of measures requiring the coordination of state and professional procedures to prevent as well as identify poor performance illustrates, realism had returned. Clinical audit, continuing professional development, linkage between appraisal and the employment contract, and assessment and support centres for doctors run jointly by the NHS and the medical profession were some of the areas addressed. Clearly for both the state and medicine there was a large agenda to take forward.

By this stage, the state's awareness that its management agenda could not simply be imposed was beginning to be matched by an awareness in medicine that the components of self-regulation, whilst remaining independent, would nonetheless have to be repositioned in order to 'fit' the regulatory component of the state. Sir Donald Irvine, then President of the GMC, observed in 1999 that 'the outstanding question is how the government's plans for clinical governance and the profession's arrangements for self-regulation are to be aligned and "docked" together to give the best results for patients' (Irvine, 1999: 1175). However, the political difficulty was that this joint approach would take time and would require painstaking negotiations. With the media enjoying a regular diet of incompetent doctor stories, such an approach, though worthy and necessary, was not regarded by the politicians as politically sufficient. Their instinct was to take action that could be seen to be taken. Such was the impetus generated by this instinct that it verged on the edge of what might be termed policy panic.

The institutional expression of this instinct was the creation of national regulatory agencies in response to the political exigencies of the moment. Although at the beginning this process was informed by a strategic view of the state's eventual destination (greater control over medicine's self-regulatory territory), this was rapidly undermined both by the scale of the political demands from public and press and by the reluctance, or inability, of the medical profession to deal with the required pace of change. NICE was the first to be established (as a Special Health Authority) in March 1999. Its functions were, first, to appraise all new technologies for their clinical and cost effectiveness and advise whether they should be in routine use in the NHS; second, to disseminate clinical guidelines based on a clear scrutiny of the scientific literature; and third, to develop and promote clinical audit. It was made very clear in the course of government consultation that the values governing the NICE's appraisal activities would be quite different from those which have traditionally informed the profession's evaluation of research and the dissemination of its views through, for example, clinical guidelines. The NICE view was that, whereas

> clinical guidelines are a comprehensive set of best practice guidance relating to the management of all aspects of a particular condition, the appraisal process will be focussed on the *value for money* of a particular intervention. (National Health Service Executive, 1999c: 19, emphasis added)

The message was that judgements about the utility of the products of medical research were no longer the sole province of clinicians. Of course, once cost-effectiveness is introduced as the dominant criterion then the economic rationing of research results in the light of the available resources must occur. NICE therefore found itself immediately visible as a rationing agent and the subject of intense controversy involving patient groups, clinicians and the pharmaceuticals regarding its judgements on drugs such as Viagra,

Relenza, Beta Interferon and Glivec. In all four cases, its initial judgement was overturned by political pressure and vividly illustrated the political dangers to the state of taking over this particular arena of medical regulation. By seeking and failing to establish its own rationalistic and economic values as the source of legitimacy for rationing decisions, NICE must have reminded the Secretary of State for Health of the benefits of covert clinical rationing through self-regulation (see e.g. Chisolm, 1999).

Whilst the NICE enabled the state to lay claim to some of the regulatory territory of clinical standard setting, the CHI (launched in April 2000, also as a Special Health Authority) was designed to provide the state with an evaluative regulatory function through its provision of 'effective systems for monitoring delivery of quality standards' (National Health Service Executive, 1999a: 6). This was to be achieved through a rolling programme of clinical governance reviews of Trusts covering 'the organisation's systems and processes for monitoring and improving services, including patient and public involvement, risk management, clinical audit, clinical effectiveness programmes, staffing and staff management, education, training and continuing personal and professional development, use of information to support clinical governance and health care delivery' (Commission for Health Improvement, 2001: 1). If the methodology of the review programme initially constituted what Day and Klein acerbically describe as 'as set of rather vacuous categories waiting to be filled' then that is probably a reflection of the fact that the regulatory ambition of the state had at this point completely outstripped the CHI's capacity to deliver (Day and Klein, 2002: 27; see also Day and Klein, 2001). But despite the implausibility of the Commission's approach, the political dynamic continued to drive it forward, so much so that in the first two years of its existence it became the fastest growing institution in the NHS with its budget doubling from £12 million in 2000–01 to £25 million in 2002–03 and its staffing numbers increasing from 180 to 300 (Day and Klein, 2002: 26).

In part this growth has been stimulated not just by the logistical needs of the invasion of medical territory, but also by the need to turn the large increase in NHS spending announced in 2002 (aiming at achieving the target of 9.4 per cent of GDP by 2008) into tangible political profit. Thus CHI is to expand its regulatory functions to monitor the use of this large investment. The government's intention is that the Commission will then have the capacity to play 'the key role ... in explaining to the public how NHS resources have been deployed and the impact they have had in improving services, raising standards and improving the health of the nation' – in other words, maximising the political profit from this investment (Department of Health, 2002b: para. 10.9). To this end, it is intended that CHI should evolve into the Commission for Healthcare Audit and Inspection (CHAI) which would 'inspect', not simply 'review' clinical governance (a significant change in nomenclature), become responsible for the 'star' system of assessing Trusts, absorb the current responsibilities of the Audit Commission, take on the regulation of the private sector from the National Care Standards Commission (NCSC) and produce an annual report on the state of the NHS (Department of Health, 2002c). Unresolved at present are the enforcement powers of CHAI: that is, the extent to which it should have the regulatory function of corrective intervention (Table 1.1). (CHI had no capacity for direct sanctions but was reliant on the Trusts themselves, the Modernisation Agency, the regional offices of the NHSE – then subsequently the Strategic Health Authorities (SHAs) – and, ultimately, the Secretary of State.)

In terms of the state–medicine relationship, the emergence of CHAI signals the desire of the state to rationalise and strengthen its hitherto disorganised probes into the territory of medical regulation. If this rationalisation is to be convincing, two other agencies established in the flurry of state actions in the wake of the Bristol, Alder Hey and related events will also need to be incorporated into a common structure: the NCAA (April 2001) and the NPSA (July 2001). Whereas CHI was designed to deal with the quality of the systems that impact on the performance of doctors, the objective of the NCAA is to identify an individual problem before it 'becomes a national scandal or a disaster'. To that end, the Authority will

> operate a new performance assessment and support service to which a doctor can be rapidly referred, where the concern about their practice will be promptly assessed, and an appropriate system devised. It will see an end to lengthy, expensive suspensions, multiple investigations of the same problem, variable local approaches and delays in actions to protect patients. (Department of Health, 2001a: 2)

However, a subsequent statement by the NCAA itself is less ambitious and more cautious, recognises the constraints under which it must operate, and seeks to contain 'unrealistic expectations that the NCAA will resolve all patient and professional concerns about doctors in difficulty'. It continues: 'We need to be clear that we are a service that can and will assist, but the responsibility still lies with the Health Authority or Trust, or with the GMC' (National Clinical Assessment Authority, 2001a: para. 6.2.2). So the NCAA can be seen as an enabling agency, which supports the regulatory process but cannot itself initiate a standard-setting, monitoring or intervention function.

In contrast to this, the NPSA falls squarely within the monitoring category of regulation (Table 1.1). Its genesis and rationale are described in *An organisation with a memory* which takes a systems approach to the analysis of adverse events, draws on the experience of other industrial sectors such as aviation, and places the responsibility for adverse events with an organisation's culture, reporting and learning systems rather than with the individual clinician (Department of Health, 2000a). Having detailed the many and variable ways in which information about adverse events in the Health Service is gathered, compiled and not integrated (e.g. the 'haphazard' reporting of incidents in the NHS, adverse reactions to drugs by spontaneous reporting by doctors to the Medicines Control Agency (MCA), complaints, and NHS and public inquiries) the report concludes that 'even where there is good evidence from high quality systems such as the Confidential Inquiries, the evidence is that implementation of lessons and recommendations is often a very slow process' (Department of Health, 2000a: para. 4.59). Such faintheartedness is not for the NPSA itself, established to coordinate the efforts of the NHS to report and learn from adverse events. Welcoming the Kennedy report on the Bristol Inquiry, its chair, Professor Rory Shaw, said, 'The Agency has been created to revolutionise patient safety in the NHS in the wake of tragic events such as those at the Bristol Royal Infirmary. We will do this by collecting information about problems, learning from them and putting into place mechanisms which actually do save lives and prevent adverse events happening in the future' (Department of Health, 2002a). Whether it was politically wise to be quite so ambitious so soon remains to be seen.

Nonetheless, it was an understandable tactic for the NPSA to adopt. The creation of national agencies as a visible response to media and public pressure has occurred in an *ad hoc* and unsystematic manner and there is, for some, an incentive to compete for the occupation of regulatory territory. The NCAA, however, takes a different line. Diplomatically reflecting on its own position, the NCAA saw itself as 'a central part of a complex jigsaw of changes to the quality framework of professional practice in the NHS. Many of these changes are not yet complete and depend on each other for their success in achieving the quality improvements' (National Clinical Assessment Authority, 2001: para. 6.2.1). In the absence of an accountability framework which binds and defines the state's various regulatory inventions one to another, and also relates them to the existing body of NHS procedures, the agencies have been obliged to negotiate 'Memoranda of Understandings' between them as the means for dividing up the regulatory territory (see e.g. National Clinical Assessment Authority, 2001b).

For the most part, the creation of new agencies as a policy response to the politicisation of medical regulation focused on the arena of performance (Table 1.1). Medical education and, in particular, junior doctors (who constitute one third of the medical workforce) have not been singled out for media attention. Nonetheless, the state took the opportunity to argue in *The NHS Plan* that the regulation of postgraduate medical education should be 'rationalised' through the creation of a Medical Education Standards Board and a new approach to medical workforce planning driven by the standards of the NSFs and 'performance managed' by NHS Trusts (Department of Health, 2000b: paras 8.28, 8.13). As Chapter 5 has shown, medical workforce planning has traditionally been within medicine's sphere of influence and an important component of its economic autonomy within the NHS (see Chapter 5). Undisturbed for decades, its review in 2000 prompted epithets such as 'Byzantine' and 'labyrinthine' as the bemused explorers of the state discovered a 'landscape of medical workforce planning ... littered with advisory groups which themselves frequently take advice from other bodies whose accountability for the results of their advice is unclear' (Department of Health, 2000c: para. 4.18). Planning was seen as fragmented, characterised by a lack of technical skills and management ownership and what amounted to a 'policy vacuum' across the NHSE and the Department (Department of Health, 2000c: para. 4.21). What was required, the review argued, was the ending of this historic anomaly and the integration of doctors into a unified system of workforce planning and funding on an equal basis with all the other health professions. Workforce Development Confederations would be the vehicle for this reform and the means for bringing medicine within the normal NHS line of management accountability.

In the regulatory arena of research, both Bristol and Alder Hey dramatically raised the issue of informed consent and illuminated the paucity of existing arrangements. Other instances soon emerged to show that, in research terms, these were not unique events but indicative, if in an extreme fashion, of the licence inherent in the traditional view of clinical autonomy. For example, the Griffiths Report into research conducted at the North Staffordshire Hospital Trust concluded that the randomised controlled trial looking at the effect of treating premature babies with continuous negative extrathoracic pressure (CNEP) ventilation instead of standard ventilation did not provide parents with adequate explanation, the opportunity for properly elicited and recorded consent, or appropriate involvement in later decision making (National Health Service Executive, West Midlands, 2000).

The state's policy response in the research arena took a number of forms. It had to address a situation characterised by a framework of ageing and obsolete legislation, a system heavily reliant on informal guidance and medical practice, and a large gap between established custom and public expectations (Chief Medical Officer, 2001: 21). In the area of organ retention alone, the CMO's report recommended: the amendment of the Human Tissue Act 1961, the Coroners Rules 1984, and the Code of Practice for post-mortems; the issuing of a standard consent form; the creation of an independent commission to oversee the return of retained organs and tissues to families who request it; and a fundamental revision of the law 'encompassing the taking, storage and use of human tissue from the living and the dead and introducing an independent system of regulatory control' (Chief Medical Officer, 2001: 38–40). This was clearly complex rule-creating work, parts of which would take some time. Whereas the setting up of the Retained Organs Commission in April 2001 to oversee the return of retained organs to families was relatively straightforward, ensuring the coordination of legal and professional criteria and procedures was not.

Even more challenging was the development of a policy appropriate to the regulation of all research in the NHS. Traditionally, research standards in the Health Service had been set and monitored by LRECs complemented, in recent years, by MRECs to deal with projects with a broad geographical constituency. Both types of committees have a mainly medical membership and constitute a state-sanctioned extension of medical self-regulation. Responding to the events at Alder Hey and elsewhere, in March 2001 the state produced the *Research governance framework for health and social care*, an elaborate bureaucratic edifice with the objective of ensuring that 'the public can have confidence in, and benefit from, health and social care research' (Department of Health, 2001b: i). Its principal components are defined in terms of the key responsibilities of the people and organisations 'accountable for the proper conduct of a study'. They are the principal investigator, the Research Ethics Committees, the research sponsor, the employing organisation, and the care organisation or professional involved in the research process. Given the ambition of the policy thus to construct an entirely new (with the exception of the Research Ethics Committees) state bureaucratic structure in the open fields of medical autonomy, there is much political spadework to be done. With what we can now recognise as a characteristic optimism of government policy making on medical regulation, the *Research governance implementation plan* sets (for NHS players) and recommends (for non-NHS players) a series of policy implementation targets (Department of Health, 2001c).

In the case of research governance, the attempted substitution of bureaucratic mechanisms for the informal operation of professional values has the effect of highlighting the extent to which medicine's NHS empire is serviced by its relationship with its colonies in the universities' medical schools and research funding agencies (e.g. the MRC). According to the implementation plan, if the policy is to work it will need to be supported by 'framework agreements' between the NHS, on the one hand, and universities engaged in medical research and funders, on the other. Universities will have to introduce research governance strategies which complement those of the NHS and funding agencies are asked to act as research sponsors (i.e. take some responsibility for the quality of the research). Behind this aspect of the policy lies the uncomfortable reality that at Alder Hey the clinical autonomy of Professor van Velzen (the doctor responsible for the unauthorised removal of children's organs) was enhanced by his employment on a joint contract which rendered him accountable, in principle, to both Trust and University and, in practice, to neither.

Having responded to the policy window of opportunity by producing a plethora of policies which lay claim to the performance, education and research arenas of medical regulation, the state then faced the problem of implementation both within the NHS itself and, in the case of research governance, between the NHS and other organisations. In all cases, the policies made reference to the contribution of the self-regulatory mechanisms of medicine and in some cases acknowledged that policy implementation was dependent on cooperation from the profession. How did medicine react to this invasion of its territory?

Medicine's divided response

Medicine is not, of course, one nation. As Rosemary Stevens observed several decades ago, 'many of the problems besetting the English professional associations of medicine have been not of authority in relationship to the government but of their own inter-relationships' (Stevens, 1966: 284). Divisions proliferate between the GMC, the 13 Medical Royal Colleges and their faculties, the specialist societies and associations, the BMA, bodies with cross-cutting membership such as the Joint Consultants Committee (JCC) and key actors such as the Postgraduate Deans. Traditionally, change in the medical profession has therefore been glacial. Before any action could be considered, 'a pattern of working relations' between the interested parties has had to be established as a result of 'the requirement imposed by regulation by professional consensus' (Stacey, 1992a: 121). This meant, as Stacey also observes, that 'the felt need to consult and consult again in order to reach consensus decisions greatly slows down the decision making process' (Stacey, 1992a: 250–1). We have already seen the effects of this relaxed approach to change management on the development and introduction of the GMC's Performance Review Procedures and the Royal Colleges' reforms of postgraduate education where a decade appears to be seen as a useful unit of planning (see Chapter 5).

However, such an approach assumes a relatively benign political context or, at least, one that has not declared open hostilities on the medical profession. The Labour government's policy onslaught challenged this assumption. It was the first time the state had attempted a direct invasion of medical territory and the profession was ill prepared. There was no strategy in place for the defence of the realm. Indeed, there was instead an awareness of the poor condition of the defences, of the limitations and fragmented character of many aspects of self-regulation. In 1995, the CMO's Review Group, with a membership drawn almost wholly from the elites of medicine, had been emphatic that 'the professional responsibility to monitor the standards of colleagues' professional performance needs to be reinforced for all doctors' (Chief Medical Officer Review Group, 1995: 3). And, with regard to the whole gamut of self-regulation, the combined view of the BMA, the Academy of Royal Colleges and the JCC was that 'whilst there is a plethora of initiatives, some less effective than others in ensuring self-regulation, there are numerous "gaps" within the existing arrangements' (BMA *et al.*, 1998: 6). In particular, over the last 20 years they regarded clinical and medical audit as having 'largely failed' due mainly to the absence of meaningful clinical outcome measures (BMA *et al.*, 1998: 4). In this view they were supported by independent research (Barnes and Hanstead, 1998; Berger, 1998; National Audit Office, 1995). Self-criticism was also present in debates at the Royal College of Physicians which commissioned a study of its functions. This found that the College was perceived 'to have so far failed to address urgent problems of self-regulation' and set out a long list of recommendations for reform (Horton, 1998).

The wave of public concern surrounding Bristol and Alder Hey thrust the limitations of self-regulation into a disconcertingly harsh political daylight. With the civil society dimension of the triangle of forces now unstable, the profession's feeling of political vulnerability was palpable. All of medicine's leading bodies no doubt accepted the sentiments of Mr Barry Jackson, then President of the Royal College of Surgeons of England, that 'the most immediate challenge for our college is the re-establishment of unequivocal confidence in the surgical profession in the eyes of the public, the media, and the politicians in the wake of recent adverse publicity' (Horton, 1998). But even assuming that the political will was there, how was the profession to coordinate both its internal and external response to public and state pressure given the historic individuality and rivalry of its regulatory bodies?

The initial response was largely to ignore this question and to assert that the principle of self-regulation constituted a necessary and sufficient guarantee of clinical quality. That is to say, that the doctor's clinical autonomy exercised in the context of accountability to their patients and their peers and appropriately supported by management is the bedrock of sound clinical standards. For example, the Central Consultants and Specialists Committee of the BMA (CCSC) began its guidance on the appraisal of senior hospital doctors with the confident assertion that 'the quality of medical practice is ultimately guaranteed by professional self-regulation, and it is therefore appropriate for the profession itself to respond to clinical governance by showing that self-regulation can work locally as well as nationally' (British Medical Association, Central Consultants and Specialists Committee, 1998: 1). The Committee then organised all its recommendations concerning performance monitoring, evaluation and correction around the single principle of peer review. By definition, in the world of self-regulation accountability to non-peers is neither necessary nor desirable because the territories of medical regulation can only be adequately administered by the professionals themselves.

Other constituent institutions in the elaborate framework of medical self-regulation took the same view and, mindful of the need to protect their particular tribal homeland, rapidly threw up what defences they could, as much against the encroachments of their medical allies as against those of the state. The aggregate product of this intense activity was a wealth of proposed initiatives, dealing with different regulatory functions, using a variety of overlapping concepts, frequently expressed in isolation from one another, and incorporating competing notions of accountability and power relationships. The impression of energy was convincing, and for a short while obscured the haphazard nature of the proposed reforms.

As one would expect given the nature of the political pressures, in terms of Table 1.1 the focus of this activity was on the regulation functions of standard setting, evaluation and intervention with regard to the performance of doctors (categories 7, 8 and 9). The dominant view was that the 13 Medical Royal Colleges and/or the specialist societies should have the responsibility for the setting of clinical standards for their members. The Colleges, in particular, had already had some experience in this area as a result of their engagement with clinical and medical audit (see e.g. Royal College of Physicians of London, 1989; Royal College of Surgeons of England, 1989). But who should do what? Some specialist societies were considerably more advanced than others in their development of relevant procedures. Senior officers of the Society of Cardiothoracic Surgeons, for example, were confident that their Society possessed the necessary database to support standard-setting procedures which, they believed, 'should go some way to restoring public confidence' in the wake of the Bristol events. The Society had, they claimed, 'democratically assumed responsibility for quality control of individual surgical practices' – a new role for any specialist society in the UK (Keogh *et al.*, 1998: 1759). However, the authors also note that other specialties are at a much earlier stage of regulation development: 'our specialty represents the tip of the iceberg in medical quality assurance, and the major challenge will be determining realistic, measurable and auditable outcomes for the other medical and surgical specialties, where poor outcomes also occur but the process is less transparent' (Keogh *et al.*, 1998: 1760).

Equally, some colleges were more experienced than others in the business of setting standards and the issuing of clinical and service guidelines. For example, in 1998 the Royal College of Anaesthetists listed 22 such guidelines and the Royal College of Obstetricians and Gynaecologists three (Royal College of Anaesthetists and Association of Anaesthetists of Great Britain and Ireland, 1998: 26–8; Royal College of Obstetricians and Gynaecologists, 1998: 2). Again, some colleges had benefited from the standard setting involved in the national confidential inquiries and others not. Given this variable level of standard-setting competence, it was unclear whether colleges could, or should, act as coordinating bodies for their respective specialist societies, particularly since the ties that bound them together were largely a matter of informal historical custom. One way forward chosen by the Royal College of Physicians was to set up a 'Clinical and Effectiveness Evaluation Unit' which, among other things, was designed to serve as a clearinghouse for guidelines relevant to its 25 medical specialties (Royal College of Physicians of London, 1999: 4).

Assuming standards could be set, the next self-regulatory question was who should monitor and evaluate them? To varying degrees, colleges could claim that they were already engaged in this arena through their monitoring of the training they accredited. One obvious avenue for their regulatory advance, should they wish to adopt it, was the enhancement of this function so that it included performance monitoring as well. Thus the Royal College of Anaesthetists' guidance on good practice contained detailed advice on the arrangements departments should have in place to ensure patient safety and the identification and management of poor performance (Royal College of Anaesthetists and the Association of Anaesthetists of Great Britain and Ireland, 1998). Working along similar lines, the Royal College of Physicians considered expanding its college network of regional advisers through the addition of a new role of 'Standards Adviser' in each Trust. This role, described as one would expect in the language of professional autonomy, was 'designed specifically to assist colleagues in matters pertaining to clinical governance and, importantly, *independent of the Trust's clinical governance machinery* although inevitably in contact with it when required' (Royal College of Physicians of London, 1999: 6, emphasis added). Where a specialist society had already developed a monitoring capacity, as had the societies for thoracic medicine, cardiology and nephrology, for example, then the assumption was that they would take the monitoring lead. Without exception, actual and proposed changes to self-regulation assumed that the monitoring and evaluation of performance would be conducted by a process of peer review with the contentious issue being the composition of the peer review team – should it be internal or external to a Trust, with or without a college involvement (Academy of Medical Royal Colleges, 1999)? In this first phase of the profession's response to regulatory challenge, flirtations did on occasions occur with the managerialist concepts of appraisal and job plans but the reflex inclusion of peer review as a dominating method in such procedures ensured that the structure of accountability remained within the orbit of medical control and quite separate from the NHS lines of accountability (e.g. British Medical Association, Central Consultants and Specialists Committee, 1998).

Moving now to the third regulatory function, if the evaluation of performance against a set of agreed standards demonstrates that a deficiency exists, what form of intervention did the profession deem appropriate? In roughly ascending order of professional severity the options available are: peer pressure, retraining, visit by a college rapid response team, suspension by employer, suspension by GMC, dismissal by employer, removal of accreditation by a college, and removal from the GMC register of qualified doctors. Much of the college-based debate initially focused on the first two categories of intervention – as is to be expected given the internalist assumptions of self-regulation. Where employers were mentioned it was generally in terms of the resources required to support the professional development needs identified rather than as a relevant contributor to the accountability process itself. Thus the Royal College of Physicians summarised the dichotomy of profession and employer by observing that 'the whole process [of clinical governance and regulation] can be seen as a dual responsibility: of the physician to maintain good standards; of management to provide adequate resources' (Royal College of Physicians of London, 1999: 8). To deal with cases of serious poor performance, and following the events at Bristol, some colleges have moved to develop rapid response teams as a more immediate form of intervention (Senate of Surgery of Great Britain and Ireland, 1998: 7). Indeed, with competitive zeal, the Royal College of Anaesthetists and the Association of Anaesthetists of Great Britain and Ireland proposed the development of ways of responding to requests for help from patients, anaesthetists, or provider Trusts 'before other statutory bodies are involved' (Royal College of Anaesthetists and the Association of Anaesthetists, 1998: 23). What they did not address, however, was what linkage there should be between a negative finding by a college investigative team and an individual doctor's college accreditation.

Watching all this diverse activity was the GMC: the body with statutory responsibility for professional standards exercised through its maintenance of the register of doctors fit to practise medicine and the power of its Professional Conduct Committee to remove a doctor from that register for 'serious professional misconduct' (General Medical Council, 1993). In addition, in 1997 it had also acquired the powers of the new Performance Review Procedure which allowed for a range of corrective actions to be taken once the nature of a doctor's poor performance had been established, ranging from retraining to, eventually, removal from the register (see Chapter 5).

From division to collaboration

The shock of the combined attack on medical territory by state, civil society and the media left the profession in disarray. Historic institutional and personal rivalries were ignited, counter attacks on the invading forces were uncoordinated and the defences appeared to be crumbling. Yet the subsequent reversal of medicine's fortunes was surprisingly swift. In part this was because the state's ambitions always vastly exceeded the logistical capacity of its managerial troops, in part because the media is an inconstant ally easily diverted by the prospect of easier spoils, and in part because medicine's instinctual identity as a professional group re-emerged when faced by a common threat to its power base. How did it succeed in regaining control of its regulatory domain?

As the body with the statutory responsibility for the standard of doctors' performance through its maintenance of the Medical Register, the GMC received the major share of the political heat as the events around Bristol, Alder Hey and elsewhere unfolded. Its strategic problem was multi-layered. On the one hand, the political demands from state and civil society required changes in the Council's ideology, structure and functions. On the other, such changes could not be achieved in isolation from the other parts of the complex institutional web of self-regulation. Traditionally, time had been used to facilitate the collaboration required by much lesser problems of reform. Now there was no time, or not much.

The GMC needed a vehicle which would enable it to demonstrate that action was being taken, to include a range of power interests from within medicine, and to construct rapidly a viable framework for self-regulation. In February 1999 the Council announced its decision that, 'to maintain their registration, all doctors must be able to demonstrate regularly that they continue to be fit to practise in their chosen field' (General Medical Council, 1999a: 1). As a political concept, 'revalidation' had been launched. The *Report of the revalidation steering group* on which this decision was based proposed a six-stage process incorporating all the three functions of governance: standards setting, monitoring and evaluation and intervention. The stages were: local profiling of performance; periodic external peer review of the profiling process; providing evidence that would lead to revalidation of the doctor's entry in the register; (and where there are concerns about a doctor's performance) local remediation; referral to the GMC performance procedures; action by the GMC on the doctor's registration (General Medical Council, 1999b). The political agenda had been set, but would it be implemented?

By taking the revalidation step the GMC signalled to both the elites of medicine and to the state that it was attempting to change its role from that of a contributor to self-regulation to one where it had a coordinating function across all parts of self-regulation. Clearly such a shift raised serious questions in the minds of the other medical elites, particularly the Royal Colleges. How would their regulatory territory and hence their power base be affected by the GMC's ambition of an explicit linkage between the governance functions of standard setting, monitoring and evaluation and intervention? What should be their contribution to the revalidation process and how should this be decided? In any case, did the Council possess the authority and legitimacy to carry through its plan particularly given that, as we shall see, it was simultaneously engaged in constitutional reform?

An important player in the ensuing drama was the AMRC, effectively a political broker of medical interests. To stimulate a debate on the way forward, the Academy issued its own consultation document on revalidation which supported the GMC's general direction but presented five organisational models of how revalidation might be implemented (Academy of Medical Royal Colleges, 1999). At the same time, the Council engaged the Medical Royal Colleges in the details of how the revalidation policy might be implemented by asking them to elaborate for their own specialties and for general practice the application of the principles contained in *Good medical practice* – the GMC's statement of the duties and responsibilities of a doctor (General Medical Council, 1995). By April 2000, discussions had progressed to the point where the Revalidation Leads Group of the AMRC (representative of all the College and Faculty interests) was able to issue the tactfully titled document *How the Royal Colleges and Faculties might contribute to the process of revalidation*, a joint statement establishing a common format for the Colleges' input to revalidation and thus a common political position on the regulatory territory which should remain in their hands (Academy of Medical Royal Colleges, 2000).

With the major issues regarding which medical institution should do what in the revalidation process both identified and under negotiation, in June 2000 the Council produced the document *Revalidating doctors* for consultation as it sought to consolidate its grip on the revalidation policy formation process (General Medical Council, 2000). Within this document we can see not only the provisionally agreed contribution of the Medical Royal Colleges and specialty associations to revalidation but also the possible contribution of the state and patients' organisations. Having seized the policy initiative within medicine, the Council now aimed to integrate into its revalidation framework the contribution of annual appraisal as part of doctors' NHS contracts, local management processes under clinical governance, and the work of bodies such as the Commission for Health Improvement (CHI) (General Medical Council, 2000: box 5). In other words, the GMC's ambition was to coordinate the policy moves of the state, as well as those of the profession: an interesting form of counter attack.

The Council's difficulty was that by this stage its political resources were very stretched. Not only was it attempting to coordinate the profession's self-regulatory response, it was also simultaneously reforming its own constitution and fitness to practise procedures – a task which engaged the same political constituencies but for different (though in the case of fitness to practise procedures, related) policy purposes. As a result, problems in one policy domain could readily impact on the support available to the GMC in the neighbouring policy arenas, and they did.

Constitutional reform of the GMC polarised the interests of medicine, the state and civil society in a way that revalidation did not because it illuminated the basic power conflict in stark numerical and structural form. The state wanted a small executive board with statutory powers to enable the GMC to become more decisive and responsive to lay concerns but the profession was divided (Dewar and Finlayson, 2001). Whilst the GMC wanted a small executive body on top with the statutory powers and a larger elected body underneath, the BMA and Colleges wanted a larger, elected body on top with the statutory powers and a smaller executive body underneath. On such matters are causes won and lost. Intense professional emotions were displayed in response to the GMC's reform proposals published in March 2001 (General Medical Council, 2001). As an indicator of the flavour of the times, one can quote an editorial in the *British Medical Journal* which opened with the apocalyptic words:

> The General Medical Council – unloved by patients, government and doctors – is close to the abyss. What might push it over the edge in the next two months is the issue of its governance, or if that doesn't get it revalidation might. The question that occurs to many is whether the council is worth all the effort necessary to save it. Might it be better to scrap what's become a dysfunctional organisation and start again? (Smith, 2001: 1196)

Unloved, perhaps, but since politics is about pragmatism, not love, progress had to be made, despite the divisions. Thus in July 2001, the Council agreed a package of constitutional reforms and in November 2001, a set of changes to its fitness to practise procedures. Following discussions between the GMC and the state, *Reform of the General Medical Council* was published for statutory consultation in May 2002 (with a joint foreword by John Hutton, Minister of State for Health, and Sir Graeme Catto, President of the GMC) and the General Medical Council (Constitution) Order 2002 was duly approved by Parliament in November of that year (Department of Health, 2002d). The Order reformed the constitution and governance of the GMC, restructured its fitness to practise procedures and enabled the implementation of revalidation. Despite all the wrangling, the future governance of the profession now rested with a GMC General Council composed of 35 members with an increased lay presence but a medical majority. With the major statutory issues thus resolved, pressure from the state on the GMC diminished and enabled it to release political capacity to deal with the continuing implementation of revalidation.

By this stage it was clear to the medical elites that revalidation should be treated as an opportunity for the profession to harness the powers of the state to its own advantage rather than as a threat to its autonomy. Having stemmed the tide of the state's policy initiatives, or perhaps more accurately waited for the state to exhaust the policy formation possibilities in the governance field, medicine could advance on its chosen front of revalidation policy implementation. In so doing, it was careful to ensure that the political needs of the state were recognised and incorporated into this process.

Appraisal was the arena where the information requirements of medicine's revalidation policy and the state's clinical governance policy met. Both policies needed information which would enable them to evaluate the performance of doctors against agreed standards and enhance or correct that performance as appropriate. One policy was driven by the profession and the other by managers. State pressure for the appraisal of doctors as a means for increasing management control over their activities had been present from the early 1990s but had made little progress. However, now the political context was different. At a superficial level, it could appear that the consequent pressures on medicine to become more accountable to managers through clinical governance have had their effect. For consultants appraisal was introduced in April 2001, for GP principals it became a contractual requirement from April 2002 reinforced by their local PCTs, and for Non-Consultant Career Grade Doctors it was launched in October 2002. But when we examine who controls the details of the appraisal policy's definition and implementation, a different picture emerges.

To take a step back, the GMC's *Revalidating doctors* policy proposal in 2000 had included a detailed consideration of how appraisal might contribute to revalidation (General Medical Council, 2000: 15–19). That view re-emerges in a joint approach to appraisal and revalidation initiated by the Department of Health and the GMC in April 2002 – described as 'an historic collaboration' – and facilitated through a joint website for doctors (Departments of Health and General Medical Council, 2002). In line with the GMC's original proposal, the basic information structure of both appraisal and revalidation is to be based on the same seven headings set out in the GMC guidance *Good medical practice* (General Medical Council, 1995). By this point, the Royal Colleges and specialist associations were well advanced in producing their specialist versions of that guidance and were establishing their claims to governance territory in terms of not only standard setting but also the monitoring and evaluation functions and, in some cases, the intervention function. For example, the RCOG stated that the 'GMC has overall responsibility for defining the revalidation process but not the mechanisms underpinning it'; furthermore that the RCOG is responsible for:

- helping the GMC to define the process in relation to our specialty
- benchmarking uniform standards across the country
- checking, by routine visits and random checks, that the procedures are occurring
- responding, with the help of senior Fellows, if a trust has concerns about an individual (Royal College of Obstetricians and Gynaecologists, 2000a).

The investment of more time and energy in standard setting meant that the Colleges were in a strong position to influence, if not take over, the state's activities in this governance arena. As we saw earlier, the NICE was established as the state's chosen vehicle in this field. It rapidly discovered that medical expertise is a scarce political resource which the profession naturally employs as a bargaining counter in its dealings with the state. The practical outcome of this power imbalance has been that NICE has commissioned standard-setting development work from the Colleges. Thus the Royal College of Physicians, for example, set up the National Collaborating Centre for Chronic Conditions (NCC-CC) in April 2001 – one of six NCCs funded by NICE to produce national guidelines and develop audit. What we have, then, is the state funding of development activities by the profession which, via revalidation, will be geared to the needs of medicine's new, improved self-regulatory apparatus.

The impetus of revalidation has also produced adaptations in the Colleges' approach to continuing medical education or, to use a more recent terminology, continuing professional development (CPD). As Clair du Boulay has observed, whereas previously the CME approach focused on the updating of medical knowledge by the individual doctor, 'the changing political climate and need to be more accountable mean that doctors now have to demonstrate that they are developing professionally and that their activities are educationally and cost effective and improve their practice' (du Boulay, 2000: 393). As a result, Colleges have an enhanced role to play because it is their responsibility to ensure the linkage between the professional needs of a doctor, the CPD available, and the process of revalidation. From being an esoteric activity of concern primarily to the individual doctor, CPD has through revalidation acquired a political significance which requires that it be managed as part of a College's maintenance of their regulatory territory. Not taking a proactive stance on CPD would mean that a College, by default, ceded that territory, or allowed the possibility of cession, to the NHS's managerial line of accountability – a politically unacceptable option.

Assuming that Colleges use CPD as the vehicle for extending their monitoring and evaluation of their members' and fellows' activities, there then arises the governance issue of intervention. Where the evaluation shows poor performance, what steps should a College take and what, if any, should be the link to an individual's College accreditation? As is discussed in Chapter 5, the Colleges' modes of intervention vary considerably (see Chapter 5). Alternatively, should they leave the intervention function to the revalidation procedure? The GMC, it would appear, does not see a conflict of interest between itself and the Colleges with regard to this governance function. Reflecting on the contribution of the Colleges to revalidation, Sir Donald Irvine, then President of the GMC, suggested a possible division of intervention labour when he wrote,

> But the real challenge and opportunity for the colleges in future lies in the further enhancement of doctors' professionalism through the meaning of membership and fellowship of the colleges themselves. With GMC re-licensure providing the statutory safety net which will deal with poorly performing or wayward doctors, the colleges have an unrestricted opportunity to show that memberships and fellowships are contemporary statements of good practice. ... It seems likely that those achieving such recognition would have it accepted for the purpose of revalidation. (Irvine, 2000: 417)

He continued, 'It is through this kind of development that the royal colleges should continue to be the dynamic growing point of professionalism in medicine, and the ultimate custodians of our basic values and standards' (Irvine, 2000: 417).

The mobilisation of the profession's many and varied forms of self-regulation within a revalidation strategy which enabled each institutional player to maintain and develop its existing regulatory territory forced the state into an immediate retreat. It could still claim that revalidation formed a part of its clinical governance policy but if, as we have seen, the profession controlled the details of standard setting, evaluation and intervention then clearly it was a fairly hollow political statement. The state could only limit medicine's regulatory counter attack if it was able to bind appraisal into the NHS's managerial line of accountability on a contractual basis. In this respect, the manoeuvring around the negotiation of the new consultant contract was of intense interest to both sides.

The state's objective was to achieve

> a stronger unambiguous framework of contractual obligations which will provide greater management control over when consultants work for the NHS and over their performance and, for the consultant, better arrangements for supporting their professional development and greater clarity and transparency about their time commitments in the NHS. (Department of Health, 2001d: para. 1)

The 'key element' of this framework was to be mandatory job planning supported by a new appraisal system which would form the basis for nominations for the proposed clinical excellence awards (Department of Health, 2001d: para. 12; on the proposed reforms to the award scheme see also Department of Health, 2001e). Given this ambition, it was not surprising that the negotiations over the contract were lengthy and arduous. Eventually, in November 2002 English and Welsh consultants rejected the new contract by two to one and specialist registrars by more than five to one. (Consultants in Scotland and Northern Ireland voted for the contract.) Their reasons for doing so were that it would have given more power to managers and that, regardless of the financial inducements of the contract, the importance of clinical autonomy as a safeguard against the changing priorities and targets of politicians had to be maintained (Smith, 2002). In the due course of time, and following the replacement of Alan Milburn with John Reid as Secretary of State for Health, the contract was renegotiated, the concerns of consultants about intrusive managerial powers addressed, more financial incentives included and in October 2003 it was accepted by the consultant body in all four UK countries (see Chapter 7). The point had been clearly made – policy implementation without the consent of doctors is not an option.

If the acute sector was one where the reality of medical power could easily block the state's implementation of regulatory policy (unless it coincided with the enhancement of self-regulation), so also was the primary care sector. Here clinical governance policy is to be delivered and managed by PCTs or through Personal Medical Services (PMS) contracts. Again, the assumption within the policy is that there is a management capacity to ensure that GPs fulfil their clinical governance obligations, a highly questionable assumption given the historic difficulties of using GMS contracts to achieve anything that general practitioners, as private suppliers of health care, do not see as in their interest. In practice, therefore, it is an unsurprising research finding that both 'managers and doctors have taken care that clinical governance be implemented mainly by GPs themselves through informal professional networks, rather than imposed through formal managerial systems or PMS contracts' (National Primary Care Research and Development Centre, 2002). Managers responsible for clinical governance in primary care reported 'that in order to engage health practitioners in quality improvement, it is essential for them [the managers] to be seen as helpful and supportive of practices' (Campbell *et al.*, 2001: 1581). Non-threatening educational activities which encouraged clinicians to engage in quality improvement were the most common form of support offered – a sensible and diplomatic option given that 41 per cent of those responsible for clinical governance implementation did not have a budget to support this task (Campbell *et al.*, 2001: 1582; see also Campbell *et al.*, 2002). Clinical governance then becomes what the medical profession in primary care wants it to be. These findings are likely to be replicated in the future given the gathering pace of the appraiser training for GPs, and thus the reality of professional control, which forms part of the joint approach to appraisal and revalidation of the Department of Health and the GMC (Departments of Health and General Medical Council, 2002).

Conclusions

In November 2002, Parliament passed the General Medical Council (Constitution) Order 2002 and brought to a close a major phase in the struggle for the territory of medical regulation. Four and a half years after the GMC's decision on the Bristol consultants on 29 May 1998 had opened an unprecedented policy window for reform of the profession, the seal was set on a revised version of the medicine–state relationship. A streamlined GMC armed with the statutory authority to implement its revalidation policy is now in position, the numerous tribes of medicine have assumed a role in that policy (though naturally still arguing about the details), and the future of self-regulation is secure. On the state side of the regulatory frontier, the new national agencies of NICE, CHAI, NCCA and NPSA stand gaunt and exposed, watchtowers for the surveillance of medicine yet uncertain of each other's bearing, let alone their relationship to the institutions of self-regulation. Meanwhile, at the grassroots managers continue to push forward with clinical governance, but starting almost from scratch they inevitably lack the resources available to self-regulation, now reinvigorated by the state-sponsored support of revalidation.

It is a far cry from the brave new world of clinical governance envisaged by *A first class service* in 1998 where, riding on a wave of public opinion and politicians' ambitions, steely eyed managers were to confront the backwoods men and women of medicine and bind their archaic mechanisms of self-regulation into the apparatus of NHS accountability. Their target, the regulation of clinical autonomy itself, was an ambitious one not attempted before. To that extent the policy makers can be forgiven for sadly underestimating the complexity of the parallel medical world within the NHS, its ability to defend its territory in depth against the probes of would be invaders and, perhaps most unexpected, its capacity to launch a convincing counter attack. There was, after all, no precedent for rapid and concerted action by the medical elites in pursuit of a common political objective. Within the profession, there was no history of the collective management of change and a long history of often-bitter infighting. Consensus had always been difficult to achieve and the initial, divided response to the state's invasion, inward looking and self-regarding, was what one might have expected.

Undoubtedly the state created its own vulnerabilities by trying to advance too far, too fast and on too broad a front. Its frantic, and largely uncoordinated, invention of agencies to deal with the emergence of new regulatory problems merely demonstrated to medicine's elites the inherent strength of their own position. To a degree, the state had no choice. Post-Bristol and Alder Hey, the level of public concern as measured on the register of media interest created a policy window that could not be ignored. A policy response had to be forthcoming. Policies, in abundance, there were. But as soon as they moved from the rarefied element of policy formation to the gritty substance of policy implementation the necessity of engagement with sources of medical expertise was unavoidable and the bargaining began.

In terms of the functions of governance, standard setting was always going to be at the heart of the profession's regulatory territory, impossible for the state to access. As soon as NICE was established it became abundantly clear that to fulfil its mandate regarding national standards it would require the cooperation of the Medical Royal Colleges and specialist societies. Cooperation there has been, but on the Colleges' terms since they control the essential knowledge resources. Monitoring and evaluation at first appeared more promising for the state, not least because through CHI these governance activities could be swiftly launched and political results obtained. But there remained the problem of intervention, who was responsible for ensuring that something happened if CHI produced negative findings about a Trust's performance? In any case, in the absence of a developed infrastructure of management-led clinical governance (an ambiguous and therefore operationally limited term) CHI, or any other non-medical agency, could not hope to penetrate the dense undergrowth of medical practice – unless the profession's elites, in their own interest, decided to facilitate that penetration.

As the *ad hoc* nature of the state's invasion became apparent, and its weaknesses thus exploitable, the medical elites did precisely that, except that through revalidation they metamorphosed the advances of the state into the gains of medicine. What had begun as a challenge to the profession ended as the means for the consolidation of its power. The resources of the state were harnessed to the needs of medicine. Somnambulant medical institutions were revitalised and new alliances forged. Undoubtedly the divisions of medicine initially inhibited this process as the rituals of historic rivalries were displayed and enacted. But the hopes of the state that these divisions would fatally undermine the profession's ability to resist were short lived.

There is something politically organic in medicine's subsequent coalescence around the concept of revalidation which defeats the slide rule of political analysis. Although the GMC had the formal lead role, it is the informal politics of medicine working through brokerage institutions such as the AMRC that made the implementation of revalidation possible. As the state discovered to its cost, there is no single locus of power in medicine with which to negotiate but rather a network of elites which form and reform as the political pressures change. The unprecedented scale of the pressure from 1998 to 2002 brought them together long enough not only to repel the invasion but also to recolonise parts of the state.

7 Medicine and the private sector

Introduction

The state's ill-starred invasion of medical territory clearly revealed the limits of its power and the extent and depth of medicine's defences. Indeed, such is the complexity of those defences that they obscured an elementary fact which the state conveniently ignored: that the NHS is but one part of medicine's estate. The majority of doctors are based either full-time (general practitioners) or part-time (consultants) in the private sector of health provision. Should the pressure on medicine's NHS territory ever become too intense, doctors always have the option of exit to the private health care provider market, secure in the knowledge that for the foreseeable future there will be a demand for their services.

In the event, this migratory option was not activated in the course of the state's assault but it remains a powerful if *sotto voce* theme in the politics of health. This is particularly so given the Labour government's new found affection for private health care and the role it ascribes to the private sector in the move towards a mixed economy of health. As the state's promises to its citizens regarding their health care rights become more ambitious, so it is having to dismantle old practices in the organisation of health care provision as it struggles to deliver those rights. In this chapter, the numerous strands of medical influence in the changing relationship between the private and public sectors of health are unravelled. First, there is the nature of the private and public markets themselves. What are the main components of the mixed economy of health care, how do they interrelate, and what are the major trends at work? Second, what are the primary dimensions of medical power in this mixed economy in terms of the systemic relationship between medicine, civil society and state; the institutional and contractual arrangements; and the regulatory procedures which govern medical accountability? Third, when analysed in terms of the main categories of the mixed economy, what are the implications for medical power of the changes now in train?

The mixed economy of health care

The health economy of the UK has always been composed of a mix of private and public financial demand, on the one hand, and private and public health care supply, on the other. Aligning these four components in a matrix produces a four category typology of the private and public sector relationships in the mixed economy of health care (Table 7.1).

The categories are:

1. *Private finance–private supply* – Private insurance companies or individuals purchasing health care from private providers.
2. *Public finance–private supply* – Publicly funded agencies (PCTs, NHS Trusts) purchasing services from the private sector: for example, GP services, waiting list initiatives, pharmaceutical supplies, laundry and catering.
3. *Private finance–public supply* – Private insurance companies and individuals purchasing health care and other services from publicly owned NHS Trusts: for example, paybeds.
4. *Public finance–public supply* – Publicly funded agencies purchasing services from publicly owned NHS Trusts.

The political significance of the typology is that it uses the concepts of health care demand and supply to identify the analytical categories which also constitute the political arenas in which the

Table 7.1 Typology of the mixed economy of health care

Health care supply	Financial demand	
	Private	Public
Private	1	2
Public	3	4

power play between medicine, the state and the market occurs. As Chapter 1 made clear, it is the ability of the medical profession to regulate the demand–supply relationship which constitutes its primary system power. Chapters 4 and 6 dealt with exercise of that power in category 4 of the typology, by far the largest and, in terms of recent political action, the most visible arena. This chapter now focuses on the other three arenas.

As a whole, the mixed economy is dynamic, varied and fluid. Just how much so is revealed by the application of the typology to a comparison of the markets of health care in 1994–95 and 2000–01 (Tables 7.2 and 7.3). While one market is dominated by the single category of public finance and public supply (acute psychiatric), in the remainder there is a distribution across two categories of the mixed economy (elective care, psychiatric rehabilitation, long-term mentally ill and learning disabled), three categories (abortions) and four categories (elderly residential long-term care). Furthermore, it is an economy where the private–public mix of markets is changing rapidly.

With the significant exception of elective surgery, between 1994–95 and 2000–01 there has been a marked redistribution of activity away from the arena of public finance–public supply and towards the arena of public finance–private supply in all sectors of the market (Table 7.4). Thus, for example, between 1994–95 and 2000–01 the private sector market share of elderly residential long-term care provision increased from 32 per cent to 56 per cent, and of learning disabled long-term care from 55 per cent to 79 per cent. Although elective surgery has so far remained immune from this general trend, there is, as we shall see shortly, every reason to suppose that the state's recent policy initiatives will diminish, if not remove, that immunity.

Within the context of this mixed economy and its general trends, the elective surgery market is important not only because of its sizeable contribution to the total value of the private sector provision of health care (Table 7.5), but also because doctors' private medical work is almost exclusively in this market and not in the others. Sensibly so, because it is in this market that the profession is able to maximise its financial and, as we shall see, its political returns. When combined, the fees of consultants in 1999 totalled £924 million – 26 per cent of the private acute sector market of which elective surgery forms the major part. Interestingly,

Table 7.2 The mixed economy of health care 1994–95

Market	Year to which relates	Data base	Category 1 Private finance–private supply (%)	Category 2 Public finance–private supply (%)	Category 3 Private finance–public supply (%)	Category 4 Public finance–public supply (%)
Elective surgery	1992–93	Cases	12	0	2	86
Elderly residential long-term care	1995	Cases	37	32	3	28
Acute psychiatric	1995	Beds	5	2	0	93
Psychiatric rehab, long-term mentally ill	1995	Beds	0	61	0	39
Long-term learning disabled	1995	Beds	0	55	0	45
Abortions	1995	Cases	36	16	0	48

Source: Laing and Buisson, 1996: table 1.3, A62.

Table 7.3 The mixed economy of health care 2000–01

Market	Year to which relates	Data base	Category 1 Private finance–private supply (%)	Category 2 Public finance–private supply (%)	Category 3 Private finance–public supply (%)	Category 4 Public finance–public supply (%)
Elective surgery	1997–98	Cases	12	1	1	86
Elderly residential long-term care	2001–02	Beds	25	56	2	17
Acute psychiatric	2001–02	Beds	5	8	0	87
Psychiatric rehab, long-term mentally ill	2001	Beds	0	73	0	26
Long-term learning disabled	2001	Beds	0	79	0	21
Abortions	2001	Cases	33	24	0	43

Source: Laing and Buisson, 2002: table 1.3.

Table 7.4 The change from public to private provision 1994–95 – 2000–01

Market	Public finance–public supply (%)		Public finance–private supply (%)	
	1994–95	2000–01	1994–95	2000–01
Elective surgery	86	86	12	12
Elderly residential long-term care	28	17	32	56
Acute psychiatric	93	87	2	8
Psychiatric rehabilitation, long-term mentally ill	39	26	61	73
Long-term learning disabled	45	21	55	79
Abortions	48	43	16	24

Sources: Laing and Buisson, 1996: table 1.3, A62; Laing and Buisson, 2002: table 1.3.

Table 7.5 Value of the major markets of the private sector supply of health care 2001–02

Market	£ million	%
Acute sector	3 530	25
Long-term care of elderly and physically disabled	8 965	63
Non-acute mental illness long-term care	389	3
Learning disabilities long-term care	1 339	9
Total	14 223	100

Source: Laing and Buisson, 2002: table 1.2.

although privately remunerated for their private work, consultants are not always physically located in the private sector when they provide the elective surgery supply. In 2000, 14 per cent of total private patient revenue was spent on the NHS provision of elective surgery ('paybeds' – the private finance–public supply category) with consultants supplying a private medical service within a publicly provided location (Laing and Buisson, 2002: table 2.9): a nice illustration of doctors' ability to move easily across the boundaries of the mixed economy.

Some doctors, it has to be said, can move across these boundaries more easily than others. General practitioners, in particular, have much less freedom than consultants to transit the boundary into the private finance–private supply category despite the fact that, unlike consultants with NHS employment contracts, they are based largely in the public finance-private supply category of health care. As private contractors, GPs supply the bulk of the NHS's primary care services. Yet only about 3 per cent of all GP consultations in the UK are privately financed: a much less significant proportion than the 13 per cent of operations privately paid for and carried out by consultants. There are several reasons for the differential presence of GPs and consultants in the private finance-private provision category and their contrasting abilities to exploit their respective private markets. Unlike their hospital colleagues, GPs are not allowed to treat patients on their NHS lists privately and so cannot use their access to the NHS market as a means for generating business. Second, a GP who sees a patient privately cannot issue an NHS prescription – which significantly increases the overall costs of private consultation. And finally, though this is now changing, there have been no insurance products designed to cover private GP consultations (Laing and Buisson, 2002: 171–2).

The dimensions of medical power in the mixed economy

Medical power in the mixed economy derives from the profession's position at the crossroads where health care demand and supply meet. Importantly for this chapter, that power operates both within and *between* the private and public categories of that economy. Immovably fixed for the last half century by custom, status and contract, consultants in particular have constituted the forum in which the relationship between demand and supply has had to be negotiated. Without them, change in the mixed economy of the politically sensitive acute sector market is difficult to achieve. By the same token, it is frequently (though not always) the case that change in one private–public category of that mixed economy will impact on another category.

The mechanisms which maintain the profession's grip on health care demand and supply act impartially across the private–public divide. Laing and Buisson observe that private sector consultants

> have a virtual monopoly of private practice because of the professionally established chain of referral from GPs to consultants, because of professional rules which prevent specialists from advertising direct to the public and because of private medical insurance rules which, with a few exceptions restrict reimbursement to treatment provided by specialists who have attained consultant status. (Laing and Buisson, 1995: A119)

In 1993 the Monopolies and Mergers Commission (MMC) determined that a 'complex monopoly' existed in the supply of private medical services, consisting of consultants who set their fees close to the BMA guidelines (Monopolies and Mergers Commission, 1993). Two years later, the BMA agreed to discontinue the publication of the guidelines, thus eliminating this source of upward pressure on consultant fees, but the structural basis of the monopoly remains intact. Its effect, as the MMC also observed, is to place the consumer, the private patient, in a weak bargaining position because the competition for consultant services is so restricted.

The economic power of consultants as the arbiters of the health care demand–supply relationship is reinforced by the political dimension to their economic activities. Successive governments have chosen to measure the extent to which the health care rights of their citizens are being delivered in various ways but the most enduring, potent and provocative measure is the time a patient has to wait for outpatient and inpatient treatment. NHS waiting lists have become an unrivalled political symbol in health care, exerting an irresistible fascination on politicians as they search for a way of capitalising on NHS spending. The most recent example is also the most impressive. *The NHS Plan* (2000) and *Delivering the NHS Plan* (2002) promise that by 2005 the maximum waiting time for an outpatient appointment will be three months and for a hospital inpatient appointment it will be six months. Furthermore, by 2008, the maximum wait for an inpatient appointment will be three months and the average wait will be half that time (Department of Health, 2000b, 2002b). To achieve these targets, spending on the NHS is projected to grow by an unprecedented rate of 7.4 per cent in real terms each year from 2002–03 to 2007–08 which, among other things, will result in 42 new hospital schemes and 15 000 more consultants and GPs.

Since waiting lists are above all a measure of the demand–supply mismatch in publicly financed health care, their continuing salience in the public debate about health gifts consultants an enviable, and thus far inexhaustible, political resource which they would be supremely irrational not to exploit to the full. Despite the close and sometimes desperate attentions of NHS middle managers over the past decade as they try to meet the latest central fiat, waiting lists remain very much a temporal extension to the private professional world of the clinician. And since many clinicians move readily between the public and private sectors of health care provision, it is inevitable that there will be an engagement between their role as arbiters of the demand–supply relationship in both sectors and their economic self-interest. Precisely what form that engagement takes has been intensely debated and generated much political heat.

In its inquiry into consultant contracts, the House of Commons Select Committee on Health noted that, 'It is argued by some that allowing NHS consultants to conduct private practice creates a system in which there are in-built perverse incentives for those consultants to allow their NHS waiting times to increase, in order to stimulate demand for their more lucrative private practice' (House of Commons Select Committee on Health, 2000: para. 48). Indeed, one vigorous proponent of this view, Professor Donald Light, has argued that consultant contracts are 'a blatant conflict of interest, an invitation to mischief' and constitute one of several government policies 'that maximise waiting times and maximise the number of patients going private' (Light, 2000: 1349). An avalanche of correspondence to the *British Medical Journal* (where Light's views were published) disagreed with his analysis. Nonetheless, what is clear is that consultants can influence the size of the waiting list by changing the admissions threshold and the operation and discharge rate (West, 1993: 59). The use of this power may be attractive in a situation where, in the absence of a price mechanism, waiting lists can denote desirability and prestige in the health care market (Pope, 1992: 79).

While the waiting list debate focuses on the demand side of the political equation of clinician power, another recurring argument regarding the division of consultant time between NHS and private work concentrates on the supply side of the same equation. Both debates highlight the political centrality of clinicians as arbiters of the demand–supply relationship and demonstrate how deeply their power is embedded in NHS practice. A key component of the 1948 concordat between medicine and state was that the national terms and conditions of service for hospital medical staff should allow all doctors to undertake private practice. As modified by the Conservative administration in 1980, for junior staff this is limited to times when they are not contracted to work for the NHS, but for consultants there is no restriction on when private work can take place. The guidance that exists is, as one would expect of a self-regulating professional group, open-ended. Consultants on whole-time or maximum part-time NHS contracts are simply advised that they should 'devote substantially the whole of their professional time to the NHS' (Department of Health, 1994a). The difference between the two contracts is that whereas consultants on whole-time contracts must not receive payments on private practice work in excess of the equivalent of 10 per cent of their gross NHS salary, those on maximum part-time contracts have no restriction on their private earnings but accept a 9 per cent reduction in their NHS salary.

For medicine, the political objective of the contract is to combine job security with the optimum professional freedom to exploit the health care market: what, in fact, one would expect of a high status and powerful professional occupation. Given that consultants' private work is remunerated on a fee-for-service basis whilst their NHS contract is based on a fixed salary, they clearly have an objective economic incentive to maximise their private earnings (assuming a demand for their service exists) – though they may, of course, choose not to respond to that incentive. But in order to take advantage of their market position consultants need flexibility within their 'labour space' and the ability to determine the timing of their service supply to the private market. What they do not need is rigorous management intervention in the planning of their clinical activities. Against this can be set the imperatives of the NHS waiting list targets. If the perennial search for particular targets is to be achieved, then managers require greater control over how consultants organise their work.

Attempts to restrict the ability of consultants to determine the balance of their private–public work as they saw fit began with the introduction of job plans in 1991 (Department of Health, 1990a). The policy is that every consultant should agree to a job plan with the chief executive which states his or her fixed commitments in detail and which can be monitored and managed. However, like many policies aimed at regulating the profession which conflict with the medical interest, its implementation has been limited. The Audit Commission's 1995 report *The doctor's tale* found that in some hospitals job plans did not exist and in many did not contain all the required information or were out of date (Audit Commission, 1995c: para. 64). In 1996 a follow-up survey revealed that a quarter of consultants did not have job plans (Audit Commission, 1996b: para. 16). Four years later, the House of Commons Health Committee commented that 'it is not possible to ascertain the extent to which consultants are failing to meet their NHS obligations because of their private work practice, because the information collected on consultants' workloads is .... currently inadequate' (House of Commons Select Committee on Health, 2000: para. 47).

Given this dearth of basic workforce information, it is then not surprising to find that the management by Trusts of their consultants' workloads is equally limited. A 1999 survey of 68 Trusts found that very few of them had sought to regulate the amount of private practice carried out by their consultants and none had refused a consultant permission to engage in secondary employment (Pay and Workforce Research, 1999). Rather, Trusts had facilitated private practice: 41 per cent had regraded full-time consultants to maximum part-time status in the previous 12 months because their private earnings had exceed the 10 per cent limit. Where action was deemed necessary because private practice was thought to be interfering with NHS commitments, it was either not taken ('too difficult') or initiated informally, usually by a senior medical colleague who might have 'unofficial words' with the offender 'behind the bike sheds' – surely the conclusive tribute to medical power. An interesting crosscutting effect of the mixed economy identified by the survey was that some Trusts with Private Patient Units (PPUs) were more concerned to provide their consultants with incentives to bring private practice into the Trust, rather than to restrict their private practice *per se*.

The ability of consultants to retain control of their professional territory in terms of their rationing function, waiting lists and the allocation of their clinical time has meant that they have also retained their central position in the mixed economy of health care. However, the acute sector market in private health care is by no means homogenous and some specialties benefit from it financially much more than others (Table 7.6). Approximately two-thirds of consultants engage in private practice with average net earnings in 1999 ranging from £75 413 for plastic surgery to £7600 for pathology. The largest part of the specialty market is anaesthetics where in 1999 consultants earned £80.4 million (20.7 per cent of the £388 million total consultant private income) followed by orthopaedics where surgeons earned £62.9 million (16.2 per cent of the consultant private market). These different levels of specialty engagement with the private sector of health care suggest that there is likely to be parallel differences in

Table 7.6 Hospital consultants (all NHS): estimated net private income by specialty, 1999

Specialty	Average private income	Number of consultants	% of all private sector consultants	Total private income £ '000s	% of total income for all specialties
Plastic surgery	75 413	169	1.2	12 745	3.3
Orthopaedics	58 959	1 067	7.5	62 909	16.2
ENT	39 763	415	2.9	16 502	4.3
Urology	39 231	358	2.5	14 045	3.6
Ophthalmology	36 325	598	4.2	21 722	5.6
General surgery	33 419	1 197	8.4	40 003	10.3
Obs and gynae	30 083	1 040	7.3	31 286	8.1
Anaesthetics	27 218	2 955	20.8	80 429	20.7
Cardio-thoracic surgery	25 786	166	1.2	4 280	1.1
Oral/maxillo facial surgery	24 353	230	1.6	5 601	1.4
Radiology	21 488	1 481	10.4	31 824	8.2
Neurosurgery	19 687	130	0.9	2 559	0.7
Psychiatry	16 658	1 896	13.4	31 584	8.1
General medicine	13 360	2 300	16.2	31 349	8.1
Pathology	7 572	174	1.2	1 318	0.2
All specialties	27 381	14 176	100	388 156	100

Sources: House of Commons Select Committee on Health, 2000: para. 38; Laing and Buisson, 2002: table 2.13.

Table 7.7 Hospital consultants (NHS England): type of contract by specialty, 1999

Specialty	Type of contract				
	Whole-time	Max part time	Part time	Honorary	All
Obs and Gynae	42	42	10	6	100
Surgery	46	43	8	3	100
Radiology	46	37	14	2	100
Anaesthetics	56	35	8	2	100
Clinical oncology	57	25	12	7	100
General medicine	58	20	12	10	100
Pathology	64	14	10	12	100
Psychiatry	73	4	17	6	100
Paediatric	78	4	12	6	100
A and E	88	7	5	0	100
All specialties	58	25	11	6	100

Source: House of Commons Select Committee on Health, 2000: para. 8.

specialty engagement with the NHS. One measure of this latter engagement is the relationship between specialty and type of NHS consultant contract (Table 7.7). Although the specialty categories of Tables 7.6 and 7.7 do not completely overlap, there is sufficient congruence for the data to show, as one might expect, that those consultants in specialties with a prominent position in the private provision of acute sector care (in terms of average salary and/or market share) are more inclined than their colleagues to opt for the maximum part-time contract with its open-ended allowance for private earnings. That a more limited contractual relationship with the NHS is associated with a closer financial relationship with the private sector is further evidenced by the MMC's finding that 49 per cent of maximum part-time consultants' earnings was from private practice (Monopolies and Mergers Commission, 1993).

The freedom of consultants to use their NHS position as the base for their activities in the private sector unfettered by over-restrictive contractual obligations has traditionally been matched by the absence of managerial constraints in their private work. Most independent acute hospitals do not employ consultants but grant practising privileges ('admitting rights') to self-employed NHS consultants working on a fee-for-service basis who may well have practising rights at more than one private hospital. In larger hospitals the grant of these privileges is on the advice of the

Medical Advisory Committee (MAC) of the hospital concerned, the arrangement creating no liability on the part of the hospital or MAC for the clinical activity of the consultant nor endowing the MAC with the power to institute auditing or monitoring systems (House of Commons Select Committee on Health, 1999: paras 24–26). In the absence of any state powers to regulate individual procedures in private establishments, this means that the quality of the clinical service provided rests with the individual consultant and, where there is a problem, with the self-regulatory procedures of the GMC. In recognising this, in its evidence to the Health Committee the Department of Health added the optimistic rider that 'it is for those using these establishments and the management to ensure quality, and with the recent growth in private health provision, market forces and competition can only improve the services offered' (House of Commons Select Committee on Health, 1999: para. 29).

However since, as we have seen, the consultant is less subject to market forces than most, this leaves the patient in a weak position, possibly subject to market failure in the quality of care delivered and armed with no recourse when pursuing a complaint except reporting the consultant to the GMC, taking him or her through the courts or utilising the uncertain investigative powers of the local Health Authority (Keen, 2000). Such is the degree of doctors' professional independence in the private sector that even the medical records of the patient remain the property of the consultant, not the hospital. The insularity of consultants is further reinforced by the lack of communication between the NHS and private hospitals. In the case of doctors suspended by NHS Trusts the Health Committee observed that

> There are gaps in information at every level. Alert letters are not made available to all registration and inspection units; neither the GMC nor the providers are always aware of why doctors have been suspended; [private] patients may be entirely ignorant of the fact they are being treated by doctors suspended from the NHS. This situation seems to us intolerable. (House of Commons Select Committee on Health, 1999: para. 113)

Intolerable perhaps, but a natural consequence of the difficulties of creating controls on the operation of medical power which span the categories of the mixed economy in health care.

Until recently, the regulation of private medicine was not a visible political issue and it remained largely protected from the immediate shock waves generated by Bristol and Alder Hey. Independent hospitals and clinics were simply obliged to register with Health Authorities under Part II of the 1984 Registered Homes Act: an Act designed to deal principally with the needs of long-term care homes and scarcely the vehicle for the vigorous monitoring of medical and surgical standards (House of Commons Select Committee on Health, 1999: paras 135–6). However, the intense debates over clinical governance in the NHS coupled with an increasing government interest in the use of private health care for NHS patients prompted a reappraisal of this hands-off approach. Accompanied by added impetus generated by the Health Committee's investigation of independent sector regulation, the 1999 consultation document *Regulating private and voluntary healthcare* led fairly swiftly to the Care Standards Act 2000 and a new regime for independent hospital regulation (Department of Health, 1999b). Under the terms of the Act, the NCSC was to be established to register, inspect and regulate care providers against national minimum standards. Created in shadow form in April 2001, the NCSC survived but briefly in the acidic waters of regulatory politics. A mere year later the government proposed its dissolution and the incorporation of its functions into the new CHAI together with those of the NHS's CHI and the Audit Commission (health value for money work). All healthcare in the UK will thus be monitored by the same body.

Moves towards self-regulation of the private sector are also being made. In 2000, the Private Practice Forum of the AMRC, working with the Independent Healthcare Association (IHA), the BMA and major insurers including BUPA and PPP Healthcare, implemented a quality framework for the private sector (Laing and Buisson, 2002: 101). In a tribute to the continuities of medical power, this framework places the responsibility for clinical governance within a private hospital with the chair of the Medical Advisory Committee.

At this stage it is too early to tell whether these novel attempts to regulate the clinical practice of doctors as they criss-cross the mixed economy of health care will have any effect. Probably more relevant to the power of medicine are the changes now occurring in the several categories of that economy and it is to this issue that we now turn.

Private finance and private supply

A postal survey by the Consumers Association found that the most important reason for respondents choosing private medical insurance (PMI) was to avoid waiting for treatment (Pay and Workforce Research, 1999: 8). Given this not unexpected finding, it is not unreasonable to argue that in the publicly financed NHS specialists engaged in private practice have an incentive to restrict the demand for acute health care, to maintain waiting lists and so divert the demand to the private sector. In the private sector, their relationship with patient demand is quite different. Here they are reimbursed on a fee-for-service basis and thus have, as the ex-policy director and current medical director of PPP Healthcare point out, 'a strong incentive to investigate and treat patients' – in other words, create demand for health care (Doyle and Bull, 2000). For those who finance private medicine (largely the PMI companies – see Table 7.8), this is unwelcome news because it may create an imbalance between subscription income and the cost of claims resulting in financial loss or higher subscriptions, though for those who privately supply health care (the clinics and hospitals) it is of course good news (more business).

In thinking through how to deal with increased consumer demand for health care provision in order to limit costs and maximise profits, insurers are obliged to recognise the imperfections of the private hospital market and the central role of doctors in maintaining those imperfections. These are, first, that there is a primacy of 'agency' relationships in that market: typically consumers do not choose the nature or location of their own treatment but as a result of the asymmetry of information between themselves and medical specialists rely on the latter as their agents to choose on their behalf.

Table 7.8 Private acute sector provision: source of revenue (%) 2001 estimates

Private Medical Insurance	65
Self-pay	22.5
NHS	7.5
Foreign and other 3rd party	5
Total	100

Source: Laing and Buisson, 2002: figure 2.4.

These agents are not sensitive to price. Second, consumption is separated from payment (hospital bills are largely paid for by third parties – the insurers), consumers are thus insulated from the financial impact of their consumption decisions, and, again, are insensitive to price. Third, it is often the case that within a given local healthcare market a specialist, or group of specialists, have a monopoly of the medical or surgical expertise available (Laing and Buisson, 2002: 76). Whatever strategy insurers adopt, therefore, they must necessarily recognise the pivotal market position of doctors and the need to sideline, incentivise, co-opt or coerce them.

In the absence of an effective price mechanism to regulate the demand–supply relationship in PMI-financed health care, insurers have adopted three main strategies. The first, and perhaps most obvious, has been to look for vertical integration of the financing and provision functions as a way of limiting the effect of consultants' agency role and getting a direct grip on provider costs. Pursuing this approach, the BUPA – the largest UK insurer with 37 per cent of the PMI-market developed its hospital division in the 1980s. However, despite its claim that its insurance and provider businesses are not integrated at the operational level, BUPA found itself the target of MMC criticism which gave a clear signal that further vertical integration would be regarded as contrary to the public interest (Monopolies and Mergers Commission, 1993). This view was reinforced by the Competition Commission in 2000 and resulted in the Secretary of State for Trade and Industry blocking BUPA's bid for the Community Hospitals Group (CHG) which would have made BUPA the largest hospital group as well as the dominant insurer. Somewhat ironically, in manoeuvring to offset the effects of an imperfect market, BUPA thus found itself criticised on the grounds that its action would reduce competition in the market for private medical services and increase prices in the PMI market (Competition Commission, 2000).

Undaunted by this setback, in the mid 1990s BUPA and Private Patients Plan (PPP) Healthcare (the second largest medical insurer with 25 per cent of the UK market) developed a second strategy based on 'preferred provider networks'. With this strategy the imperfections of the market are addressed by insurers seeking to 'direct' subscribers to the most efficient hospitals by offering them discounted insurance schemes. The selected hospitals are then able to spread their fixed costs over a larger volume of activity, aggregate claims costs are reduced through a fall in average treatment costs and insurers are in the position of being able to seek further efficiencies by demanding larger discounts from the participating hospitals. Subscriber demand and efficient hospital supply are thus brought together. Or at least, that is the theory. As ever, the success of any strategy concerning the demand–supply relationship in health care is dependent on the key role of consultants at the nexus of that relationship.

Laing and Buisson identify two consultant referral effects which can undermine the network strategy and may take place at the same time. What they term 'consultant drag' can occur where consultants do not bother to find out whether a patient has opted for a network product and refer all patients to network hospitals with the result that non-network patients are 'dragged' into the network hospitals. Second, a 'counter-drag' effect can occur where consultants, resentful of being forced to use one particular hospital and wishing to maintain the viability of others, decide to send patients to non-network hospitals. 'Counter-drag' can also occur where continued referrals to a local networked hospital leads to a rise in waiting time and consultants consequently choose to refer to a non-networked hospital with a lower waiting time (Laing and Buisson, 2002: 152). Recognising consultants' ability to make or break the network strategy, in 1997 BUPA initiated its Consultant Partnership scheme which offered consultants a 5 per cent bonus (subsequently increased to 10 per cent) on referrals to BUPA's network hospitals. Both the Hospital Consultants and Specialists Association and the BMA advised their members not to join the scheme on the grounds that it restricts consultants' freedom of choice and is not in the best interests of patient care. Undeterred, by 2002 about 7180 consultants had joined the Partnership accounting for 60–65 per cent of all BUPA covered inpatient and day case medical procedures (Laing and Buisson, 2002: 155).

The use of incentives to encourage consultants to participate in the network schemes recognises the centrality of their clinical decision-making power and therefore enhances the probability that this particular insurer strategy for dealing with the imperfections of the market will work. A third strategy, that of managed care, has enjoyed less success. In its developed American form, managed care incorporates a number of elements designed to take market power away from the clinician and give it to the health care purchasing agency, managers and administrators (Fairfield *et al.*, 1997; Iglehart, 1994). Through the use of detailed guidelines, decisions about diagnosis and treatment (and therefore about the demand for and supply of health care) are transferred from the medical to the managerial province and doctors are obliged to work within a framework not of their making (though it will have been constructed with the help of other doctors). Attempts to introduce managed care in the UK's private sector have been limited and have encountered considerable professional opposition. In 1992, BUPA introduced clinical pre-authorisation (where the insurer makes a judgement about whether a consultant's proposed treatment for a patient is appropriate) for psychiatric care, ITU, rehabilitation and oncology. However, its proposed introduction of pre-authorisation for hysterectomies provoked fierce opposition from the London Consultants' Association and the BMA (Ferriman, 1999). Unlike their American medical colleagues, most British consultants are protected from the vagaries of the market by the warm embrace of state employment as they transit from one category of the mixed economy to another. Given this secure bargaining position, they are highly unlikely to concede vital clinical territory to the ambitions of managed care unless their own interests are simultaneously advanced.

Public finance and private supply

The policies of the Labour government on both the mixed economy of health care and the position of medicine within that mixed economy have changed significantly since its return to office in 1997. Initially, the political rhetoric and actions of the Secretary of State for Health, Frank Dobson, were very much 'old Labour': anti-private health care and, following the events at Bristol Royal Infirmary in 1998, anti-doctor. Immediately on its arrival, the new administration issued guidance that NHS agencies should only purchase services from the independent sector as a last resort and subject to clearance from the regional office of the NHSE (Department of Health, 1997b). This was followed in 1999 by the abolition of GP Fundholding (a small but significant source of private hospital revenue from the NHS) and the decision to exclude private health care from the new clinical governance framework being set up for the NHS. Other fiscal measures chipped away at the private sector – such as the abolition in the July 1997 budget of tax relief on PMI policies for over 60-year olds.

None of this particularly bothered the insurers and private hospitals. The measures were aimed at restricting a demand for private medical services which rested largely with a robust PMI sector (NHS revenue composed only 7.5 per cent of total demand for the private acute sector – Table 7.7). Potentially rather more threatening were Labour moves on the supply side. Negotiations on a new consultant contract began in the latter part of 1998 with the clear intention on the government side of bringing consultants into the mainstream of NHS managerial control. If the government was successful, the private sector would find the flexibility of its consultant medical workforce much reduced.

In the event, the political logic of the state's broader ambitions for the NHS conspired to re-emphasise consultant power, undermine the state's bargaining position *vis-à-vis* the profession, and redefine aspects of the dynamic within the mixed economy. Propelled by voter disillusionment with the NHS, traditionally a Labour policy stronghold, in 2000 the Prime Minister announced unprecedented increases in Health Service expenditure in order to bring overall public and private spending on health care to 7.6 per cent of GDP. As we saw earlier, that ambition was incorporated into *The NHS Plan* along with a raft of waiting-list targets. That left the obvious question of where the extra capacity to deliver these targets was to come from. In the longer term it was assumed that more doctors and nurses would be trained and hospitals built. But what of the short- to medium-term? In an historic shift of Labour Party health policy, the Plan opened up the issue of active private sector engagement: 'The time has now come for the NHS to engage more constructively with the private sector, and at the same time make more of its expertise available to employers throughout the country' (Department of Health, 2000b: para. 11.1). Among the policy avenues mentioned were Diagnostic and Treatment Centres (DTCs) to be developed jointly with the private sector, new public–private partnerships, and the NHS Local Improvement Finance Trust (NHS Lift), to improve primary care premises in England.

The replacement of Frank Dobson by Alan Milburn as Secretary of State for Health in October 1999 had signalled a symbolic shift from old to 'new Labour' thinking in health policy formation. Unburdened by the 'statist' ideological legacy of Labour's past, Milburn could happily set about the task of harnessing private sector capacity to Labour's new Health Service project. In his evidence to the Health Committee's investigation of the role of the private sector in the NHS, the Secretary of State maintained that 'shortages of capacity in the public sector constituted the principal factor prompting him to make greater use of the private sector ... His approach was both to develop greater capacity in the NHS and to make targeted use of the private sector while this was coming on stream' (House of Commons Select Committee on Health, 2002: para. 14). In fact, as each new policy idea was added to the list of types of engagement between the NHS and the mixed economy of health care, so it became apparent that a much more fundamental shift was taking place than Milburn's pragmatic views had suggested.

First formal recognition that the new approach to the private sector was bearing fruit came in November 2000 with the joint publication by the Department of Health and the IHA of a concordat between the public and private sectors which began: 'There should be no organisational or ideological barriers to the delivery of high quality healthcare free at the point of delivery to those who need it, when they need it. The Government has entered into this concordat with the Independent Health Care Association to set out the parameters for a partnership between the NHS and private and voluntary health care providers' (Department of Health and Independent Healthcare Association, 2000: para. 1.1). Although in the first instance work was to focus on the areas of elective care, critical care and intermediate care, it was also intended that 'there should be a move towards a more collaborative and proactive approach to long term capacity planning' Department of Health and Independent Healthcare Association, 2000: para. 3.1). Subsequent guidance reinforced this message and required 'the whole range of local independent providers' to have representation in the capacity planning process (Department of Health, 2001f). £20 million was allocated to the initiative in 2001–02 rising to £40 million in 2002–03.

Before inquiring further into the policy avenues down which the Labour government's new-found enthusiasm for the private sector has taken it, we need to pause and reflect on the position of the consultants in this unfolding scenario. The elementary political fact is that as the monopoly suppliers of medical expertise in both the public and private sectors, the interests of consultants would need to be included in whatever policy deals were reached between the politicians and the private sector elite. Yet in *The NHS Plan*, for example, we find that New Labour's penchant for muscular management found expression in the proposal that there should be a ban on private practice for the first seven years of a newly appointed consultant's contract. Such an aggressive approach failed to recognise that the political significance of the pivotal position of consultants in the mixed economy of health care was considerably enhanced by the state's need to make that economy work in pursuit of its expansionist aims, particularly when the success or failure of those aims was to be measured in terms of waiting list targets. Even allowing for the post-Bristol halo effect, the state's optimism regarding its ability to bring consultants to heel through a new contract which tied appraisal, job plans and activity into a seamless management sequence was bordering on the foolhardy. Effectively, by its exclusive reliance on the new contract negotiations as the only means for ensuring the integration of consultants into the political jigsaw of a revamped public–private relationship in health, the state was boxing itself into a corner.

However, the gathering pace of the push towards a mixed economy NHS tended to regard the position of doctors in the jigsaw as a lower order tactical issue, to be resolved as and when. In a series of speeches Milburn outlined the policy moves being made and the rationale behind them. Two examples provide an indication of the extent of the policy ambition. At the NHS Confederation in July 2002 he listed the following initiatives:

> We have taken a hard look at where the private sector can help. First, using spare capacity in the private sector, such as in private hospitals, to perform operations on NHS patients. Second, getting private sector management to run some of the new stand-alone surgery centres [Diagnostic Treatment Centres] our Manifesto commits us to building and which will specialise in precisely those procedures where private hospitals have some expertise. Third, extending PFI beyond the hospital sector where it has already helped deliver the biggest hospital building programme the NHS has ever seen into new Public Private Partnerships in primary care, social services and the provision of equipment. And fourth, using private sector management expertise such as

in the provision of IT systems. It is around these four activities that we will force a new relationship between the NHS and the private sector. (House of Commons Select Committee on Health, 2002: para. 7)

And at an international gathering in May 2002 to discuss the proposed new Foundation Trusts, the Secretary of State approvingly quoted 'the more diverse European model of provision' and linked the private sector with the theme of patient choice in the NHS.

> For patient choice to thrive it needs a different environment. One in which there is greater plurality in local services which have the freedom to innovate and respond to patient needs. It is an explicit objective of our reforms therefore to encourage greater diversity in provision and more choice for patients. Hence new providers from overseas being brought into this country – alongside greater use of existing private sector providers – to expand capacity for NHS patients. Primary care trusts having the explicit freedom to purchase care from the most appropriate provider – be they public, private or voluntary. (Department of Health, 2002e)

The concept of the market is not mentioned, but that is where the logic of these policy developments naturally leads.

Within this drive for a greater plurality of services across the mixed economy, two policy initiatives in particular engage with the medical interest: DTCs and overseas doctors. The objective of the DTC policy is to separate routine elective surgery from emergency or complex work, offer patients fast-track care, and thus reduce hospital waiting lists. Centres may be run by the NHS, the private sector, or through partnerships between public and private organisations. Of their very nature, DTCs are designed to serve the needs of local NHS health economies and, in the absence of any external intervention, are inevitably dependent on the goodwill of the local monopoly suppliers: the consultants. As the demand–supply brokers of the local economy of elective care, consultants therefore find themselves in even greater demand and in the position of making choices regarding the disposal of their scarce skills and time not only between the NHS and their existing private work but also between these and the DTCs. In this situation, the plurality of the demand-side institutions has increased but that of the supply-side workforce has not.

In a direct attempt to address that supply-side inflexibility (and its consequent effect of increased consultant bargaining power), the state has introduced a policy of recruiting, or attempting to recruit, overseas doctors particularly within the framework of the DTC scheme. Published in June 2002, *Growing capacity* sets out the format of a centrally managed 'international establishment pro-gramme'. The policy aim is to draw on spare capacity in other health care systems to create 'a new sector in health care provision in England' based on independently managed and operated units, and staffed by an overseas medical workforce (Department of Health, 2002f). A defining feature of this document is its emphasis on the role of the market in terms of 'market entry', 'market management' and 'market framework' indicating a clear desire on the part of the state to use international market forces as a means for reducing its reliance on, and hence the power of, UK doctors. In his closing speech to the NHS Confederation 2002 annual conference, Milburn maintained that overseas clinical teams would become 'a permanent feature' of the NHS (Health Service Journal, 2002: 12).

However, as one might expect, the early signs were that the pol-icy would not have an easy ride from the medical profession. At the local level, there has been a mixed reaction. On the one hand, there are indications that consultants resent the intrusion of over-seas doctors, the impact of their activities on NHS waiting lists and, *ipso facto*, the likely knock-on effect of a reduction of demand for consultants' private practice (Limb, 2002). On the other, the remuneration requirements of overseas doctors working for a north west London DTC has already had an effect on the local health market and resulted in an increase in the level of fees con-sultants are able to charge for their services beyond the normal BUPA guidelines (Stephenson, 2003). As the dimensions of the mixed economy expand to include the international market, so consultants may find themselves able to escape from the fee limita-tions of the UK private sector. Meanwhile, at the national level, the GMC and Medical Royal Colleges are keen to ensure that their regulatory oversight is maintained and that overseas doctors go through the appropriate procedures of professional accredita-tion prior to engaging in UK-based employment.

In secondary care, the state's intense preoccupation with the contribution of private health care to the reduction of NHS waiting lists serves to increase medical power. In primary care, that preoccupation and the media interest which accompanies it is, by comparison, much less intense and so also is the political advantage that the profession can accrue as a result. On the surface there would, nonetheless, seem to be political mileage to be gained. *The NHS plan* set the target that by 2004 patients will be able to see a GP within 48 hours. At the same time, to achieve that ambition a second target of increasing the supply of GPs by an extra 2000 (headcount) above the 1999 level by 2004 was also set. As private sector businesses which contract to deliver a primary care service for the state (what the Audit Commission describes as 'a unique private/public partnership' – Audit Commission, 2002: para. 21), GPs' negotiating power is partially dependent on the extent that the state's requirement for their services exceeds the available supply. There is every indication that the current shortage of GPs will continue.

To achieve the 2004 target of increased GP numbers requires an average annual growth of 1.4 per cent and a wastage rate from general practice at or below the current level. However, the Audit Commission notes that current growth has fallen to 0.9 per cent which means that by 2004 there will only be 628 extra GPs, not the 2000 aimed for. Furthermore, the whole-time equivalent (WTE) number of GPs is in any case likely to be lower because an increasing proportion works part-time (Audit Commission, 2002: para. 133). This pessimistic (in terms of state targets) scenario reflects a historic trend of slow growth in the GP workforce. While the number of hospital medical and dental staff grew by 36 per cent between 1990/91 and 1998/99, the number of GPs grew by only 5 per cent over the same period (Audit Commission, 2002: para. 193). Since it is reasonable to assume that the demand for GP services has expanded at least at the same rate as that for secondary care, this means that the scarcity value and hence the market power of GPs has increased disproportionately when compared to that of their consultant colleagues. However, their ability to exploit this market position is considerably less than that of hospital doctors.

Bound as they are by the terms of the national GP contract, GPs lack the flexibility enjoyed by their consultant colleagues in translating their theoretical market advantage into tangible economic benefits. Furthermore, in the absence of a private insurance market for primary medical care and given the lack of appetite of the public for the self-pay option in primary care, the state remains their only substantial customer (Laing and Buisson, 2002: chapter 4). As the difficulties experienced by the Medicentre chain in its attempt to establish commercially viable walk-in clinics has demonstrated, the development of this part of the private care market is an uphill task (Shamash, 2002). GPs are therefore likely to remain firmly ensconced in the publicly financed and privately supplied category of the mixed economy rather than move seamlessly between categories as do consultants.

Private finance and public supply

For the majority of their private patient treatments, consultants are obliged to move not only between categories of the mixed economy of health care (from public–public to private–private) but also between physical locations (from NHS Trust to private hospital). If that physical location could remain the same, then clearly both the convenience and efficiency of consultants would be optimised. The private finance and public supply category of the mixed economy provides the means for achieving that enviable combination through the treatment of privately funded patients in NHS paybeds. In the 1970s, the NHS controlled well over 40 per cent of the private patient market (Table 7.9). However, the hostility of the 1975–79 Labour government towards paybeds coupled with the building of new private hospitals caused a rapid decline in that market share. Despite the arrival of the Margaret Thatcher's Conservative government in 1979 the slide was not checked until 1990 when a low point of 11 per cent was reached. Thereafter, the benefits of the 1988

Table 7.9 NHS private patient revenue and NHS market share of total private patient revenue, by selected years, 1972–2001

Year	NHS private income (£ million)	NHS market share (%)
1972	14	48
1982	54	18
1992	164	14
2001*	351	13

Note: * estimate
Source: Laing and Buisson, 2002: table 2.9.

Health and Medicines Act (which greatly extended the freedom of Health Authorities and Trusts to earn revenue from private patients) fed through in terms of refurbished PPUs and an improving market share which peaked at 15.7 per cent in 1997 before falling back in the late 1990s. That retreat was largely caused by adverse market conditions including the exclusion of many NHS PPUs from the major insurers' partnership networks. The latter has in turn had the effect of making the inclusion of PPUs in Private Finance Initiative (PFI) hospital projects less attractive.

Apart from a matter of convenience, it is doubtful whether the precise location for the delivery of their private practice is of great moment to consultants. Indeed, it is arguable that some consultants may not wish the Trust to whom they are contracted to have information on all their private activity and prefer to spread their work among several providers of private facilities. They are, afterall, essentially peripatetic providers of a public and a private medical service. Neither the demand for their service nor their private income is likely to change radically simply because their location alters. What matters is the abiding strength of their position in the mixed economy market and their ability to translate that position into political capital. For example, when in order to expand its cardiac surgery service the University College London Hospitals NHS Trust purchased the privately owned Heart Hospital in 2001, a third of the unit's 95 beds were reserved for private patients in order to protect the consultant interest. The Trust's chief executive commented: 'We have started from the proposition that the existing consultants will want to bring the same number of private patients in' (Gulland, 2001a: 358). Where else would one start?

Conclusions

In a letter to the *British Medical Journal* in December 2001, a specialist registrar in trauma and orthopaedics summed up the state's fundamental political dilemma in its ambition to use the mixed economy to deliver more NHS-financed health care:

> Alan Milburn's latest proposals for an increased use of the private sector for NHS patients flies in the face of his argument that newly qualified consultants will not be able to work in the private sector for seven years after attaining that status.

Or will he just bend the rules so that he can have his cake and eat it? (Ashford, 2001)

In the absence of an effective international labour market of doctors, any expansion of any part of the UK mixed economy of health care where the skills of doctors are required is dependent on a supply of medical expertise largely employed by the NHS. Thus any contractual restriction on the flow of that expertise will reduce the flexibility of the supply side of the mixed economy and diminish the ability of the NHS to draw on the spare capacity of the private sector. Yet if the state is to make the optimum use of the NHS medical workforce it employs and pays for, then it must seek to manage doctors directly.

Viewed from the other side of the political fence, medicine's power in the mixed economy is based on doctors' arbitration of the demand–supply relationship across all categories of that economy. To the extent that they accept constraints on that freedom, their market power is diminished. In its reply to the Health Committee's report on the private sector the government made clear that it did, indeed, want 'to have its cake and eat it':

> The [proposed] new contract introduces a stronger, unambiguous framework of contractual obligations, with greater management control over when consultants work for the NHS and over their performance. It will tackle any perceived or actual conflict of interest between consultants' work for the NHS and their own private work ... There will also be a new set of contractual provisions governing the relationship between consultants' NHS commitments and any private practice they undertake. (Department of Health, 2002g: 6)

Greater contractual control would enable NHS managers to intervene in doctors' labour space and thus reduce, if not eliminate, their market dominance of the demand–supply relationship.

It was for this reason that the negotiations over the new consultant contract were so intense and protracted and why in England (where the majority of private practice takes place) it was ultimately rejected by consultants and, resoundingly, by specialist registrars in November 2002 (Smith, 2002; see Chapter 6). (Consultants in Scotland and Northern Ireland where private practice is much less developed voted for the contract.) Afterall, no sensible political actor knowingly undermines his own power base. Further evidence of state failure to curb the mixed economy freedoms of doctors came with the announcement in January 2003 that the government had abandoned plans to restrict consultants' private practice: what Andrew Foster, NHS Director of Human Resources, admitted was a 'major pull back' from its initial position (Health Service Journal, 2003). This realistic assessment was then incorporated in a much revised national contract, accepted by the consultant body in October 2003, where private practice was reinstated as a normal part of consultant activity (Department of Health, 2003c: Schedules 9 and 10).

As defeats go, it was a serious one because so much else depended on this particular battle. Driven by the imperatives of waiting lists, in the space of two years the Labour government had reversed its traditional antipathy towards private medicine and formally embraced it through the concordat with the independent sector. By so doing, the state not only injected a fresh dynamic into the mixed economy of health care but also provided the private sector with a welcome respectability. For consultants, a reinvigorated pluralism in health care financing and supply could only be good news since it re-emphasised their centrality in the mixed economy and, in the absence of the new contract, state dependence on their cooperation. As yet it is unclear how far that dependence will be mitigated by a significant increase in the supply of overseas medical expertise. What is clear is that on the whole it is not in the interest of the two-thirds of consultants engaged in private practice to facilitate that increase.

If the state has had to recognise the intransigence of medical power in the public–private category of the mixed economy, so also have the insurers in the private–private category. Moves towards the vertical integration of the finance and provider functions have been blocked by the state, managed care has received a frosty reception from the medical profession and preferred provider networks have worked to the extent that consultants have received extra incentives to use their market power to make it work. Like the state, the private sector insurers and hospitals are reliant on a professional group which, when under pressure, has the option of exiting to another category of the mixed economy.

In responding to these pressures, the medical profession does not, of course, act as one. For the most part, GPs remain locked in the public–private category while the majority of consultants are able to transit and benefit from the mixed economy at will. Moreover, within the consultant group there are wide inter-specialty differences in the rewards to be gained from private practice and hence different motivations guiding consultants' contractual relationship with the NHS. However, such differences only have political significance to the extent that they can be exploited and, as yet, neither state nor private sector has discovered a formula which would do so.

8 Conclusions – the new politics of medicine

Introduction

At one level, the politics of medicine today appear to be characterised by instability, conflict and change. Patients are more demanding and less easily satisfied, managers have been armed with the weapons of clinical governance by the aggressive policies of politicians, and doctors are busy reforming their procedures of self-regulation under the watchful eye of the media. Civil society, the state and the profession seem to have abandoned the certainties of yesteryear for a new form of much less predictable political engagement. Yet at another, more significant level it has been argued in this book that the fundamental tenets of the triangle of political forces driven by the problem of citizenship remain firmly in place (Figure 1.1), that the political dependencies and benefits of that arrangement may have been redefined but not replaced, and that continuities in the power relationships between the major players are the dominant feature of the politics of medicine.

This means that at the mesa- and micro-levels of analysis we see a reformulation of the relationship between the principal actors of patients, managers, politicians and doctors but not a significant redistribution of power between them, dependent as that distribution is on the systemic logic of the triangle of forces. Behind this interpretation lies a view of the adaptability of the many roles and institutions involved in the politics of medicine and of the prevalence of incremental political change therein. Ministerial and media claims that seismic events are taking place in and around the medical profession have to be viewed with scepticism, as do the claims of some medical politicians that the culture of medicine has been suddenly reborn as a symbiotic partnership with the empowered patient. This is not to say that medicine is not highly politicised. Clearly it is. But the politics is geared to the preservation of medical power in a new and more acceptable form, rather than its dismemberment and redistribution.

This book has drawn largely on contemporary evidence. But in so doing it has sought to demonstrate that the impact of Bristol, Alder Hey, Shipman and other events on the politics of medicine forms part of a long-term dynamic at work in this domain. In this context, this chapter reviews the evidence and its implications for the future. Given the frenetic political activity in this arena over the past few years, what is the nature of the balance struck between the political needs of civil society, medicine and the state? Are the numerous adjustments made to accommodate these needs likely to provide a sustainable model for the future, or shall we shortly witness another round of citizen and state assaults on the medical fortress? These questions are addressed in terms of the power relationships between doctors, on the one hand, and patients, managers, politicians and, a necessary question, other doctors, on the other.

Doctors and patients

Discussions of the micro-level power relationship between doctors and patients are frequently characterised by analytical and moral certainties which fail to recognise both the fluidity of that relationship and the extent to which it is inevitably embedded in, and constrained by, broader social and political structures. On the one hand, the strength of the traditional paternalistic relationship is documented in terms of the asymmetric knowledge exchange between doctors and patients, the professional as privileged expert, and the ability of the doctor to employ various techniques of communicative dominance. Alongside this view can be positioned the medicalisation thesis regarding the apparently inevitable capacity of the discipline to absorb ever more areas of social deviancy into the realm of medical diagnosis and therapy. On the other hand, arguing with equal certainty, are writers who maintain that expert knowledge systems are increasingly permeable, questioned and questionable; that citizens are able to mount significant epistemic challenges to medicine through the creation of their own life-worlds aided, for example, by their membership of self-help groups; and that the rise of complementary and alternative medicine demonstrates the emergence of a discerning health consumer. Alongside this view can be placed the idea of patients as rational actors negotiating with reflexive aplomb the risks and uncertainties of post-modern society.

The various interpretations of the challenges to medical hegemony in the doctor–patient relationship are enlivened by a vibrant brand of health consumer advocacy so that the road to patient empowerment becomes not so much an analytical conclusion as a moral imperative. Notions of the autonomous patient, the expert patient and the resourceful patient have developed to the point where they constitute a political lobby in their own right. Their rigid assumptions regarding the inherently beneficial effect of patient empowerment (in all its various permutations) are best seen as a significant ideological component of the current health care debate rather than as a useful insight into how the doctor–patient relationship is actually evolving. For it is clear that there is, and always has been, much in this relationship that springs from the affective domain of human behaviour: on both sides of the equation. Fears, likes and dislikes are as much a part of the interactive compound as is the rational thinking of the informed citizen or the concerned professional. Indeed, it may be, as one reflective health consumer advocate points out, that 'The reality for most patients is not that we want to be in control of decision making. Maybe we just don't want to feel like everything is out of our control. Illness or injury can be frightening, especially when it affects our children' (Bastian, 2003: 1278; see also Sweet, 2003). Equally, doctors are not automatons but sentient actors who will, for example, talk more to the patients with whom they identify and resent patients who come armed with internet information (Cooper and Roter, 2002; Wilson, 1999).

The importance of affect in the psychological relationship of doctors and patients also signals a neglected aspect of their social relationship: that patients need doctors not just because of the knowledge they possess but also because patients want access to 'a healing class' which, as Blumenthal points out, 'offers hope that an apparently incurable illness may be overcome and that comfort is available when cure is not' (Blumenthal, 2002: 533). Afterall, historically, the distinctive competence of the medical profession is a function of the rise of biological science in the late nineteenth and twentieth centuries. Prior to that it was the profession's social identity as the healing class which was the prime source of its power; a power which 'derives not from any validated distinctive competence but from something more enduring and deeply rooted: a primal urge to project onto some group the power to heal' (Blumenthal, 2002: 533). If we accept this argument then the profession's control of knowledge as a political resource is supplemented by the advantage that there exists a social need for trust to be invested in a particular group as the chosen vehicle for dealing with crucial life, and death issues.

The political implication of this interpretation is that a sole reliance on rational interpretations of the doctor–patient relationship as the means for understanding the operation of medical power at the micro level is seriously flawed. Public trust in doctors (the practical expression of their professional legitimacy and the basis of their utility as arbiters of the demand–supply relationship in health care) is likely to be influenced by factors which lie beyond a rational calculation of how well doctors are, or are not, regulating their knowledge territory. Nor is it simply a question of deciding where the knowledge territory of doctors ends and that of patients (expert or otherwise) begins. What Bristol, Alder Hey and, more recently, the Cyril Isaacs Investigation have illuminated is the powerful cultural forces which surround the ownership of the body, dormant for decades but now re-emerging as the hegemony of medical science is steadily weakened (Department of Health, 2003b). From a position where body parts were regularly stored for possible future medical research with scant, if any, regard for the proprieties of consent, both profession and state have been obliged to amend their procedures significantly in recognition of the cultural requirements of civil society (see e.g. Department of Health, 2002j; Royal College of Pathologists, 2000).

Emotional, rational and cultural factors have combined to demand a redefinition of the doctor and patient roles. However, this is not a linear process: the pressures are not acting in a single direction. Nor do they necessarily imply a loss of power by doctors in their relationship with patients. More demanding patients may mean that they are potentially more, rather than less, dependent on the doctor. There is no reason to suppose that these demands cannot be met by the adaptation of the physician's role in ways which enhance rather than diminish its power. The increased availability of information on the internet, frequently conflicting and unreliable, may mean that patients are more reliant on a professional who can sift, advise and, most importantly, decide on a particular course of action. For some patients the traditional doctor role will be sufficient, for others an emphasis on consultation and information brokerage may be more appropriate. Provided that the medical profession is sufficiently flexible to adapt to these pressures, its status and legitimacy as 'the healing class' will be maintained.

The reformulation of the doctor–patient relationship at the micro-level is taking place within an ideological context which favours an extension of patient power. Over the past two decades, market and democratic values in the Health Service have been much promoted by the state though a variety of policy initiatives ranging from the Conservatives' internal market and patient choice to Labour's Patient Forums. In terms of the policy discourse at least, the patient interest is the driving political force in the NHS. So much so that it could be argued that this must in time have its own effect on the doctor–patient relationship. Across the board, formal health policy invariably incorporates the ambition of patient involvement, be this in the sphere of the Modernisation Programme or clinical service delivery. However, when we look beyond the florid rhetoric to the mesa-level political gains of patients, no significant power shifts are discernible. We find ourselves instead in the land of symbolic policy making where the objective of the state is to obtain the maximum legitimating effect for its policies with the minimum of power concessions. As an ideological theme, 'patient empowerment' is a valuable political resource which is being exploited to the full.

The political reality is nonetheless that the policy networks of health consumers, when compared to those of doctors, are fragmented, weak and largely tangential to the health policy community. The long and tangled history of the policy to replace the CHCs with the Patient Advocacy and Liaison Services (PALS) and the Patient and Public Involvement Forums drew strong criticism of the Department of Health from the Health Committee of the House of Commons (House of Commons Select Committee on Health, 2003). It was clearly a policy with a low priority at the Department and its cavalier treatment illustrates the inability of health consumer groups (unlike the medical lobby) to exercise a decisive influence on the policy-making process where their interests are at stake. Equally, there is no indication that the state either wishes or needs to forge a new, high level, political alliance with the interests of civil society in this policy field. Such an alliance would create a new dependency that the state can do without. Instead, the state is happy to continue manufacturing new forms of sponsored consumerism where it stays in control of the policy agenda.

Doctors and managers

Opening a conference at the Royal College of Physicians on the doctor–patient relationship, the Chief Medical Officer, Professor Liam Donaldson, exhorted his audience: 'We have to see ourselves as the servants of the patient, not their masters' (Macdonald, 2003). As we have seen, such a bold statement can be readily included in the new discourse of doctor and patient without resulting in a destabilisation of the underlying power relationship. Rather, it constitutes the rhetorical component of a new version of the doctor's dominant role. However, it is unlikely that the discourse of the doctor–manager relationship, despite all the regularly rehearsed overtures of peace and friendship, would include such an extreme statement. The basis of the power relationship is quite different, and therefore so also is the language.

In 1920 Sir George Newman, the first chief medical officer at the Ministry of Health, speaking to the BMA said:

> The state has seen in the profession a body insistent on the privacy and individuality of its work, the sanctity of its traditions and the freedoms of its engagements. The profession has seen in the state an organisation apparently devoted to the infringement of these traditions and incapable of putting anything worthy in their place. It has feared the imposition of some cast iron system, which might in practice make the practitioner of medicine servile, dependent and fettered. (Edwards and Marshall, 2003: 116)

But who would impose such a system? Beginning with the Griffiths reforms launched in 1983, the state has sought to use managers as the political instruments to re-engineer its macro-level relationship with medicine. As the ability of the medical profession to manage the widening gap between citizen's expectations and the NHS supply of health care came under serious strain, politicians came to the conclusion that more muscular systems of accountability were required to ensure that doctors carried out their part of the concordat between medicine and state. If doctors were unable to match patient demand with the available resources, they must be enabled to do so. As if by serendipity, the state found available both an ideological and an operational answer to its problem.

The rise of the New Right in British politics in the early 1980s and the emergence of the New Public Management approach to the problems of welfare delivery combined to challenge the indispensability of professionals in general and doctors in particular. With their emphasis on the restorative powers of the market, the importance of public choice and the need to remove the dead hand of 'producer capture', the New Right values challenged the traditional reliance of the state on the medical profession as the primary vehicle for the resolving the demand–supply mismatch in health care. At the same time, the new managerialism branded bureaucracy as inflexible, professionalism as anachronistically paternalistic and the tradition of bureau-professionalism in the Health Service as obsolete (Clarke and Newman, 1997). Armed with its own language of organisational efficiency and performance measurement, managerialism promised a one-stop political solution to the apparently intractable problems of the NHS through the use of population needs identification, commissioning, contracts and the optimal use of organisational resources. Within this brave new world, patients were to become health consumers and doctors a cog in the organisational machine.

Seduced by the obvious attractions of these blandishments, the state progressively abandoned its erstwhile partner, the medical profession, and rapidly promoted the new class of NHS managers in its political affections. Convinced by the ambition of the new managerialism, the state came to believe that doctors would be obliged to become part of the new management-led systems of accountability. For their part doctors naturally felt abandoned and aggrieved – though, in a sense, judging by the comments of Sir George Newman, they should not have been entirely surprised.

With the internal market reforms of the early 1990s, managers were given the responsibility for ensuring that doctors formed part of the corporate effort to fulfil the contractual agreements with commissioning agencies and, following the introduction of the

Patient's Charter, the Charter's targets. The policy assumed that doctors would adjust their clinical decision making and their waiting lists (the primary rationing mechanism) to suit the needs of their employing organisation. If implemented, such a shift would have meant a reduction in the doctors' clinical and political autonomy and an enhancement of managerial influence over traditionally medical political territory. In the rarefied world of the internal market policy, a redistribution of power over the demand–supply relationship in health care would occur because commissioners would define the population's health care needs, managers would arrange for the services to meet those needs, and doctors would ensure that the patients they saw and the conditions they treated (the met demand) equalled the needs identified by the commissioners. Despite a marked change in the policy discourse, this logic remained intact under the subsequent Labour governments.

What effect did the policy have on the balance of power between doctors and managers? Some analysts took the policy literally and argued that the plethora of new management structures would inevitably translate into an erosion of medical autonomy (e.g. Flynn, 1992). Others were more sceptical and saw a successful rearguard action by the profession in operation (Exworthy, 1998; Pollitt, 1993). When measured in terms of the key rationing territory of waiting lists, it is clear that the urgings from managers regarding the penalties for non-compliance had an effect on clinician behaviour. But was this an indicator of increased managerial power or an illustration of how the medical profession can adapt its rationing function and the personal and professional benefits that accrue from its operation? By 1996 the maximum waiting list time for an operation had been reduced to 18 months. This is quite long enough a period to allow consultants to use waiting lists for their traditional political purposes: achieving status (longer waiting lists equal demand for valued service) and private income (diversion of waiting list patients into private practice). So it can be argued that this flexibility allowed doctors to accommodate the demands of managers at little or no cost to themselves.

Senior clinicians were quite happy to use the new language and practices of commissioning and contracting provided they retained control of their clinical decision making. The fact that the policy discourse has changed did not mean there had been a shift in the balance of power between doctors and managers. In their ethnographic study of the contracting process in Wales between 1993 and 1995, Griffiths and Hughes show how the public discourse and procedures of contracting were paralleled by a private realm of bilateral understandings, often arising from longstanding relationships between senior managers and clinical professionals. It was through these social networks and the trust they embodied that a dialogue could be facilitated where the professional commitment to patient care could be combined with the requirement to manage limited resources, usually on the clinicians' terms. There is little doubt who was ultimately in control since, as Griffiths and Hughes observe, managers 'remain reliant on medical expertise and clinical care in the hospitals, and are heavily dependent on the co-operation of clinical professionals within the contracting teams to manage problems at the interface'. As in the past, doctors were able to use their cultural authority to resist real change (Griffiths and Hughes, 2000: 220).

In any case, managers had, and have, few direct levers of control over clinicians' activity. They can badger, argue and perhaps persuade but they have no ultimate sanction: consultants cannot be sacked unless they are deserted by their colleagues and GPs are independent contractors. It has to be remembered that although currently employed and/or funded by the state, doctors always have the option of market exit into the private economy of health care. Nor did the Conservative reforms give managers a template against which to measure clinicians' activity and performance; the much vaunted job plans for consultants introduced in the early 1990s rarely moved beyond the cosmetic adjustments required to demonstrate consistency with the relevant NHSE circular; medical audit remained firmly within medicine's professional orbit; and management's influence over the new, local distinction awards for consultants was limited. Yet, at the same time, managers were very vulnerable to consultant pressure. A vote of no confidence in a manager was a clear signal that their employment with a particular Trust was about to be terminated.

Managers' tenure as the politicians' favourites was shortlived. By 1995 Stephen Dorrell, then Secretary of State for Health, was ordering that management costs should be reduced by 5 per cent and that there should be 'less grey suits and more white coats'. Thereafter, the reduction of management numbers game became almost as complex, and, as a political football, at times as salient, as that of waiting lists. As a measure of political exposure the message was clear: managers would find themselves sidelined and scapegoated by politicians as and when convenient. And with an inexorable logic, as the star of managers faded so their ability to implement policies in the face of medical opposition at the local level diminished: if their political masters would not support them, who would?

Despite a fluctuating relationship between doctors and politicians, the downward trend in managers' political credit begun in the mid-1990s has never been reversed. It is now axiomatic in the NHS discourse that 'management costs' should always be reduced. New Labour set itself a target of a £1 billion management saving over five years from 1997. The Department of Health's 2001 report on expenditure predicted that '£1 billion that would otherwise be spent on bureaucracy will be freed up for patient care' (Department of Health, 2001j; quoted by Appleby, 2001). Managers are numerically and politically expendable. Their marginality is illustrated by their virtual absence from the consultation document on the future NHS workforce *A health service of all the talents* where just one paragraph was devoted to managerial staff (Department of Health, 2001h). At the same time, of course, the planned numbers of doctors is ever increasing.

As the instruments of the state's attempts to re-engineer its relationship with the medical profession, managers have never been entirely welcomed by doctors though their degree of hostility tends to vary according to how seriously a particular government is seeking to corral medical freedoms. With the launching of the clinical governance policy in 1998 and the attempted invasion of medicine's self-regulatory domain, relations between doctors and managers deteriorated to a new low. Even those clinicians formally engaged in hospital management (medical directors and clinical directors) found this latest incursion a bit much. A survey of the views of doctors and managers on the doctor–manager relationship conducted in 2002 found a marked divergence of opinion. Whilst chief executives were resolutely optimistic about the relationship, clinical directors were highly disaffected with many holding negative opinions about managers' capabilities, the respective balance of power and influence between managers and clinicians, and the prospects for improved relations (Davies *et al.*, 2003). As a result, it is not surprising that, as the CHI highlighted in its first annual report on the state of the NHS, recruiting doctors to take up management roles is as difficult as it ever was (Mooney, 2003). On the whole, the culture of medicine does not value management activities, or values them negatively, and therefore engages with them in only occasional and peripheral fashion.

Proof, if proof were needed, of the resilience of the doctor–manager antipathy came in 2002 with the rejection by the consultant body of England and Wales of the proposed consultant contract – laboriously negotiated over a two-year period (consultants in Scotland and Northern Ireland voted for the contract). The government's stated objective in the new contract was increased managerial control over the work, performance and professional development of consultants (Department of Health, 2001d). Job planning, appraisal and the newly proposed clinical excellence awards were to be linked together in a seamless web of managerial accountability. It was not to be. There was what Richard Smith, editor of *British Medical Journal*, described as 'a collapse of trust' by doctors in managers and government. Doctors, he observed, 'don't want to be good corporate citizens. They want to be valued professionals' (Smith, 2003: 1098). As their rejection of the contract showed, they have the power to make the choice. Thus when in October the following year the UK consultant body accepted a national contract it was a much revised one that recognised the reality of medical power: the financial incentives had been increased, the continuing right to private practice incorporated and managerial control diminished (Department of Health, 2003c). The chairman of the BMA's consultants' committee, Dr Paul Miller, commented that the major sticking point of the original contract was the 'excessive and inappropriate managerial control' over when and how consultants should work. Under the new deal, he said, the focus would be on 'joint planning where consultants and managers sit down and work out what needs to be done' (Kmietowicz, 2003: 945) – a phrase interestingly evocative of the Cogwheel consensus style of NHS administration of the 1970s.

Doctors and politicians

In October 2002, the Institute of Healthcare Management issued a press release entitled 'NHS managers keep quiet rather than tell it as it is'. A poll of over 400 NHS senior managers conducted in 2002 found that 51 per cent, from board level down to heads of departments, felt unable to raise concerns about the NHS, or their own organisation, for fear of recrimination (Institute of Healthcare Management, 2002). The results of the survey symbolise the difference between managers and doctors. Doctors have an independent power base; managers do not. It is this power base with which politicians are obliged to engage.

In so doing, politicians are constrained by the fact that, ultimately, they need doctors more than doctors need them. At the level of the political system, politicians have to deliver the health care rights due to civil society regularly and promptly. If they do not, they will be heavily penalised by the electorate. Doctors, likewise, have to fulfil the terms of their social contract with citizens and maintain public trust by ensuring that their professional care is delivered to an appropriate standard. This then enables them to manage the relationship between the demand for and the supply of publicly funded health care on behalf of the state. However, if politicians withdraw support for the medical profession doctors will survive: they have their own institutions and alternative markets. If doctors withdraw support for politicians, on the other hand, there is no alternative to them as the purveyors of health care.

The illusions of policy and the prominence of the political theatre serve to obscure this elementary, but dominating, fact of British political life. Policy formation has always been much easier than policy implementation, and this is particularly true of health policy. Many factors intervene between the policy wish and its fulfilment, not least those power groups on whom its implementation is dependent (Gunn, 1978). In a sense, all this is saying is that the construction of policy is but one part of a much larger political process, including its implementation, and that the significance (and insignificance) of particular policies should always be judged within that context. But for politicians, this interpretation is over-sophisticated and unhelpful. What they require is a policy that enables them to demonstrate they are responding to a political problem today, regardless of whether the policy may, or may not, be subsequently implemented. As one acute observer of the British political scene, Harold Wilson, observed: 'a week's a long time in politics'.

The mobilisation of civil society opinion hostile to doctors in the wake of Bristol, Alder Hey, Shipman and a host of other events presented the state with both a problem and, it seemed, an opportunity. How could it develop a policy response in a territory of regulation which was large, complex and where it had no presence? Yet given the level of public concern something had to be done and to be seen to be done. In the event, the rapid emergence of the clinical governance policy suggests that the Labour government was considering the reformulation of the relationship between state and medicine prior to the breaking of the Bristol story. Thereafter, it sought to surf the wave of public concern as the means for making rapid policy inroads into medicine's self-regulatory domain. Policies duly emerged and institutions were born with a profligate disregard for either inter-policy logic or their chances of implementation. It was simply assumed that somehow the existing structures of medical self-regulation would fall into line or be forced into line by strong-willed managers. New acronyms abounded. NICE, CHI (or CHAI as it now is, a symbol of institutional instability), NCCA and NPSA were added to the lexicon of NHS regulatory agencies in a flurry of bureaucratic enthusiasm.

Some analysts have ascribed considerable political significance to these initiatives, effectively confusing form with substance. Thus Harrison, quoting the example of NICE, considers that 'state co-option of medical elites has been a key element in government strategy. Whilst members of the medical profession, and professional organisations, indeed play a key role in the construction of clinical guidelines, this enterprise is now conducted under the supervision of state agencies' (Harrison and Dowswell, 2002: 226). This interpretation ignores the reality of knowledge control, the basis of medical power. It only makes political sense for the medical profession to trade with the state in its control of medical knowledge if there is thereby an exchange which results in a net political gain for the profession. Otherwise inaction (or where necessary obfuscation) is the rational option. Cooperation with state agencies and the process of policy implementation therefore takes place on medicine's terms, albeit cloaked in the discourse of bureaucratic rationality. Although for a brief period the wave of scepticism about doctors rendered the profession both objectively and subjectively vulnerable, the moment soon passed and the logic of medicine's epistemological power reasserted itself. Meanwhile, the state had exposed itself through its proclamation of ambitious policy objectives for the governance of doctors and was now, suddenly, more than ever dependent on the profession for the realisation of those objectives. It was an opportunity not to be missed and the re-colonisation by medicine of parts of the health care state are now in train. Private interest government is alive and well.

Nowhere is this imbalance of power between doctors and politicians more apparent than in the policy of clinical governance. Here the policy assumption was that the mechanisms of self-regulation would be harnessed in support of a management driven system of clinical accountability. In the event, the reverse has happened and the profession has used its own policy of revalidation as the means for harnessing the details of employer-provided appraisal to the needs of the GMC. Technically it remains unclear how the accountability lines of revalidation and clinical governance interconnect (Riley, 2003). In practice what is clear is that it is the regulatory bodies of medicine that control the primary governance functions in this performance arena (Table 1.1). The Royal Colleges and specialist associations set and monitor the performance standards for the different specialties and the GMC provides the means of corrective intervention or, should it prove necessary, the ultimate sanction of removal of the license to practise and registration. Nothing an employing Trust could introduce could remotely parallel or substitute for this arrangement.

Even a cursory perusal of medicine's sprawling regulatory empire demonstrates why this is the case and why the state's assault on the territory of the profession was sublime in its ambition and hopeless in its quest. When analysed in terms of knowledge control functions, that territory spans the full range from research through education to performance. Its institutions have grown up slowly and idiosyncratically, adapting themselves to the local terrain and to those political dwellings surrounding them. Their procedural interrelationships are complex and, to the outsider, virtually impenetrable. In the case of education, for example, GMC, medical schools, universities, Royal Colleges, specialty advisory committees, postgraduate deans and other lesser lights combine to transport the medical novice along the elaborate path of professional initiation. How could politicians hope to penetrate this institutional jungle without the assistance of native guides – who, in any case, might prove hostile or untrustworthy? Thus the abrasive intentions of *The NHS plan* for a 'rationalisation' of postgraduate medical education through the creation of a Medical Education Standards Board (a policy redolent with the language of the managerial state) has since been translated through the good offices of the Academy of Medical Royal Colleges into a body, the Postgraduate Medical Education and Training Board, which faithfully incorporates all the existing interests of medical postgraduate education in an appropriate hierarchy of state-financed committees (Department of Health, 2002k). The formal accountability of the Board may be to the Secretary of State for Health but its operation and power lie entirely in the hands of the profession.

Within the triangle of forces, the political weakness of the state and its dependence on medicine is, in part, a result of the profession's historic ability to limit the supply of new doctors through the instruments of workforce planning. The ratio of doctors per head of population is considerably lower in the UK than in most other European countries. In the politics of the British welfare state, therefore, doctors constitute a scarce economic and political resource. Of late, politicians have sought to redress this imbalance through the good offices of the private health care market. With the signing of the Concordat between the NHS and the private sector in October 2000 (Department of Health and the Independent Healthcare Association, 2000), the state took a symbolic step in encouraging new flows of medical labour into the Health Service arena. This was reinforced by its *Growing capacity* guidance which explicitly encouraged the growth of a 'genuinely additional workforce capacity' through the use of medical staff from overseas in the proposed independent DTCs (Department of Health, 2002f). In May 2003 at a meeting with managers from private US, European and South African companies bidding to run the DTCs, the Prime Minister Tony Blair made it clear that he wanted to expose the whole of the NHS to outside competition: 'We are anxious to ensure that this is the start of opening up the whole of the NHS supply system so that we end up with a situation where the state is the enabler, it is the regulator, but not always the provider' (Gulland, 2003).

If the operation of medical workforce choice through the mechanisms of the international health care market reduces the dependence of politicians and state on the existing supply of doctors, a change in the macro-balance of power will have taken place. One would not expect the medical profession to connive in a negation of its own power. As yet, there is little reason for medical concern or action on this front. Although the Concordat resulted in some increase in privately provided NHS acute work, this largely consisted of spot purchasing to solve short-term local problems rather than in any strategic reconfiguration based on long-term planning (Goddard and Sussex, 2002; Moore, 2003). In the case of the DTCs, obtaining access to an international supply of new doctors has proved less straightforward than the state had hoped. International health care companies are alert to the political sensitivities of investment in this field, the GMC and Royal Colleges have to be on board in order to validate the credentials of overseas doctors, and the possible impact on the training and provision of NHS services is a developing issue. Above all, local consultants, on whose cooperation the success of DTCs rests, may decide that the injection of a new source of medical supply into their local health economy would jeopardise their private practice by reducing patient demand. Alternatively, if consultants are themselves recruited to DTCs there are already indications that they could use it to enhance their private sector practice through judicious use of the referrals system (Carlisle, 2003a).

The ability of consultants to move seamlessly across the divisions of the mixed economy, plying their trade where they will, secure with their NHS maximum part-time contract yet free to choose the time and place of their private sector work, is both a fundamental feature of the Health Service and an indicator of medical power. Despite the politicians' rhetoric about the increased freedoms available to the NHS it is the doctors who exercise the choices which determine the demand–supply relationship in health care in both the public and private sectors. As the politicians move to embrace the private sector as a new ally, so they are likely to become more aware of the arrangements already in place between the private sector and medicine, of the accommodations to the medical interest embedded in those arrangements and of private health care's desire that their existing markets should not be destabilised by impetuous state interventions. What at present remains the unknown quantity is the possible contribution in the longer term of a new and substantial international supply of doctors. As yet the institutions of UK medicine do not perceive this as a threat and it will be interesting to see how they mobilise their international networks should they come to do so.

Doctors and doctors

Reflecting on the Conservative's internal market reforms, Klein observed that 'the most important consequences of the NHS reforms may thus be not so much that they changed the balance of power between clinicians and managers but that they prompted the medical profession to take pre-emptive action to prevent such a shift taking place' (Klein, 1995: 325). Since then, of course, rather more has been required of the medical profession in terms of both the manner and content of its response to challenges to its power from patients, managers and politicians. Those challenges have, to varying degrees, affected the full range of both the regulatory functions of standard setting, monitoring and intervention and the arenas of research, education and performance. As a result, none of the many institutions of medicine have fully escaped the consequences of politicisation, though some have proved considerably more adroit than others in fashioning a suitable response.

Given that their capacity for concerted defence against sustained attack had never before been tested, the numerous tribes of medicine found themselves on a sharp political learning curve. Over time, historic epistemological divisions coupled with overlapping regulatory functions had produced a mosaic of governance which, to the newly mobilised military planners of the profession's elites, posed large organisational and logistical problems. Who was to defend what and in alliance with whom? If the state could exploit these uncertainties it could, perhaps, divide and rule.

At the heart of the political storm raised by Bristol Royal Infirmary and subsequent events sat the GMC. As the body with the statutory responsibility for maintaining the public's trust in doctors, the Council felt the full force of the destabilisation of the contract between medicine and civil society. Not only was its own position under threat but also the principle of self-regulation itself. Broadly speaking, its response took two forms: an internal reform of its constitution and procedures and, more significantly for the future politics of the profession, an external re-alignment of its relationship with the other elites of medicine in pursuit of the policy of revalidation. The internal reform introduced on 1 July 2003 was big enough and the largest since the GMC's establishment in 1858. Membership of the Council dropped from 104 members to 35 and the proportion of lay members increased from 24 per cent to 40 per cent. Much energy and aggression was expended on the debate surrounding the reform and the government took a view, but essentially the reform was an internal and relatively esoteric matter – though of course of large symbolic importance in demonstrating the profession's willingness to adapt to the needs of modern governance.

However, the revalidation policy where, from Spring 2005, doctors will be required to demonstrate their fitness to practise on a five-year basis, raised sensitive and novel issues of inter-institutional power and territorial compass. Prior to agreement on revalidation and in the heady atmosphere of the immediate post-Bristol situation, the different Medical Royal Colleges, specialist societies, and groups such as the JCC had produced a disparate array of idiosyncratic proposals for regulatory reform reflecting the traditional separation between them. Precisely how there was a shift from this fragmented approach to the single policy of GMC-led revalidation to which all were signed up is unclear. Undoubtedly the medical elites recognised they must bury their differences in the common interest of survival and undoubtedly, also, brokerage institutions such as the AMRC played a significant role in facilitating the birth of a revalidation consensus which recognised the regulatory contribution of diverse institutions. More generally, one is left with the impression that the profession has evolved a set of informal rules and networks for harnessing a collaborative political effort; rules that could be invoked anew should the occasion arise.

Suspicions remain. In his annual review in 2001, the President of the Royal College of Physicians, Professor Sir George Alberti, expressed 'a major concern ... that the power of the College is slowly but surely being eroded as the government and the GMC lay claim to more and more territory' (Alberti, 2001). Some institutions of medicine are more gripped by regulatory ambition than others. In May 2003 the Society of Cardiothoracic Surgeons announced that it would publish star-ratings for its members based on death rates on the operating table: a very specific and public form of professional accountability. In large part this decision was a consequence of promises made by the Society in response to recommendations of the Bristol Inquiry. Nonetheless, it immediately ran into fierce opposition from the Royal College of Surgeons and the BMA's CCSC (Carlisle, 2003b).

The BMA, in particular, has found the now established emphasis on regulation in the relationship between medicine, civil society and state less than helpful to its position in the hierarchy of medical elites. Unlike the other major institutions of medicine it is only tangentially in the business of knowledge control. Rather, it assumes that doctors have that control and then benefits from the consequent professional leverage in its trade union role of negotiating for economic gains and advantages. Now that the activities of knowledge control through the functions of standard setting, monitoring and intervention are a central part of the continuing negotiations between profession and state, the BMA finds itself on the margins of the key debates. Connections can be made between the occupational focus of the Association and the regulatory focus of the GMC and Royal Colleges. Appraisal, for example, is a key area where the regulation of performance meets the conditions of employment and the CCSC has been very involved in the evolution of a procedure which suits the management needs of clinical governance and the professional needs of revalidation. However, the BMA has yet to turn this linkage to sustained political advantage. Indeed, in the negotiations over the consultant contract, of which appraisal formed a part, the Association misread the views of its members and in 2002 found its joint proposals with the government roundly rejected by the English consultants. Subsequent negotiations secured a much amended consultant contract acceptable to the Association's membership but the reputational damage to the BMA leadership remained.

While the politicisation of self-regulation has produced a general recognition among medicine's leading players that a continuing reform of its regulatory procedures is a necessary facet of the profession's politics over the next few years, there is disagreement over precisely how far and how fast that reform should travel, particularly now that revalidation has apparently taken the sting out of the state's approach. The profession has become accustomed to its new political visibility and this, combined with the easing of the pressure from civil society and state, is allowing the re-emergence of its traditional internal divisions and the likely slowing of the pace of reform.

Conclusions

The new politics of medicine are a product of rapid institutional mobilisation in response to intense and sustained pressure from civil society and state. Medical institutions and individuals with little experience of high-profile, media-driven politics found themselves having to evolve new policies, formulate new alliances within the profession and adopt a new patient centred political discourse. However, although on the policy surface much has changed with patients empowered to make the choices they will, managers equipped with a range of governance procedures, and politicians able to point to a host of state-run regulatory agencies, beneath the waves the political currents of the triangle of forces between medicine, civil society and state continue to exercise their dominating influence. What we have, then, is superficial change in the context of the continuities of medical power.

Undoubtedly the triangle of forces was destabilised for a while and perhaps even the medical elites believed the rhetoric of the politicians. But what has emerged from the contest is a strengthened profession and a weakened state. In the most propitious of political circumstances in the immediate post-Bristol period, the state launched a full-scale attack on the medical stronghold and failed to make any significant gains. Apparently lacking appropriate intelligence regarding the logistical complexity of the territory it was attempting to seize, the state overstretched itself and became vulnerable to policy counter attack. It succeeded in demonstrating only that its shock troops, the managers, were little more than paper tigers. Meanwhile the profession, although initially dismayed by the permeability of its position on a variety of issues, rediscovered its traditional capacity to coalesce when under attack. As it rapidly rebuilt its self-regulatory defences as the prelude for its own offensive, medicine demonstrated to itself and to its opponents its resilience and its ability for self-reinvention.

Save only for the BMA, the net internal effect has been a strengthening of the major institutional elites at the expense of the rank and file. The expansion of the self-regulatory territory through revalidation and other measures has created an internal competition for the control of this politically lucrative new realm. Specialist societies and Royal Colleges vie with each other in their stated ambitions to regulate their memberships. At the same time, and building on this activity, the institutions of medicine are looking outward to the new agencies of state regulation such as NICE and CHAI where there are opportunities for colonisation. As the state's expectations of these bodies continues to expand, so they are obliged to negotiate with the self-regulatory apparatus of medicine in order to recruit the medical expertise necessary to obtain quick political results. Thus is created a dependency on medicine from which the profession can hope to gain new forms of access and influence over the health policy community.

There is no indication that that community considers it has any serious alternative to a continuing engagement with the profession. No other power group has the ability to facilitate or to impede the implementation of policy so effectively. Patients' organisations are too fragmented to offer a meaningful counter balance to those of medicine, and are only useful for legitimating pre-conceived policies. Managers are regarded by the state as expendable, part of the necessary theatre of policy presentation but lacking real political weight.

Nor is there any reason to suppose that the interdependence between medicine and state will alter significantly in the foreseeable future. As the endgame of the NHS is played out and new ways are sought to deal with the demand–supply mismatch in health care, the move to a mixed economy will simply illuminate the profession's existing influence in the private sector. It will become apparent that governance issues regarding public trust and the protection of patients can, once again, more readily be dealt with by the mechanisms of self-regulation than by the invention of new state agencies. Thus it is from the very nature of medicine's organic politics that the continuities of its power derive.

References

Academy of Medical Royal Colleges (1999) *Proposals for revalidation.* London: Academy of Medical Royal Colleges.

Academy of Medical Royal Colleges, Revalidation Leads Group of the Academy of Medical Royal Colleges (2000) *How the Royal Colleges and Faculties might contribute to the process of revalidation.* London: Academy of Medical Royal Colleges.

Adams, L. (1998) *In the public interest: developing a strategy for public participation in the NHS.* London: NHS Confederation.

Alberti, G. (2001) Message from the President, in Royal College of Physicians, *Annual Review 2001.* London: Royal College of Physicians.

Allsop, J., Baggott, R. and Jones, K. (2002) Health consumer groups and the national policy process, in R. Saras and A. Petersen (eds), *Consuming health* (pp. 28–65). London: Routledge.

Allsop, J. and Mulcahy, L. (1996) *Regulating medical work: formal and informal controls.* Buckingham: Open University Press.

Altenstetter, C. (1989) Hospital planners and medical professionals in the Federal Republic of Germany, in G. Freddi and J.W. Björkman (eds), *Controlling medical professionals: the comparative politics of health governance.* London: Sage.

Anderson, E. and Anderson, P. (1987) General practitioners and alternative medicine. *Journal of the Royal College of General Practitioners,* 37: 52–5.

Appleby, J. (2001) Cut and run. *Health Service Journal,* 5 July 33.

Armstrong, D. (1982) The doctor–patient relationship: 1930–80, in P. Wright and A. Treacher (eds), *The problem of medical knowledge* (pp. 109–22). Edinburgh: Edinburgh University Press.

Arntson, P. and Droge, D. (1987) Social support in self-help groups, in T. Albrecht and M. Adelman (eds), *Communicating social support.* Beverley Hills: Sage.

Ashcroft, R. and Pfeffer, N. (2001) Ethics behind closed doors: do research ethics committees need secrecy? *British Medical Journal,* 322: 1294.

Ashford, R. (2001) Who will do these operations in the private sector? *British Medical Journal.* Electronic letter. 20 December. http://bmj.com/cgi/eletters/323/7320/1025.

Association of Community Health Councils for England and Wales (1999) *Commission on representing the public interest in the Health Service.* London: Association of Community Health Councils for England and Wales.

Audit Commission (1993) *Practice makes perfect: the role of the Family Health Service Authority.* London: HMSO.

Audit Commission (1994) *Trusting in the future.* London: HMSO.

Audit Commission (1995a) *Briefing on GP Fundholding.* London: HMSO.

Audit Commission (1995b) *A price on their heads – measuring management costs in NHS Trusts.* London: HMSO.

Audit Commission (1995c) *The doctors' tale. The work of hospital doctors in England and Wales.* London: HMSO.

Audit Commission (1996a) *What the doctor ordered. A study of GP Fundholders in England and Wales.* London: HMSO.

Audit Commission (1996b) *The doctors' tale continued. The audits of hospital medical staffing.* London: HMSO.

Audit Commission (2002) *A focus on general practice in England.* London: Audit Commission.

Bale, J. (2001) New laws will stop 'shocking' organ removal. *The Times* 29 January: 6.

Barnes, R. and Hanstead, K. (1998) Check-up time. *Health Service Journal*, 21 May: 26–7.

Barnes, M. (1999) Users as citizens: collective action and the local governance of welfare. *Social Policy and Administration*, 33(1): 73–90.

Bastian, H. (2003) Just how demanding can we get until we blow it? *British Medical Journal*, 326: 1277–78.

Beck, U. (1992) *Risk society: towards a new modernity.* London: Sage.

Bendall, C. (1994) *Standard operating procedures for local research ethics committees – comments and examples.* London: McKenna and Co.

Benfari, R.C., Eaker, E. and Stoll, J.G. (1981) Behavioral interventions and compliance to treatment regimens. *American Review of Public Health*, 2: 431–71.

Berger, A. (1998) Action on clinical audit. *British Medical Journal*, 316: 1893–94.

Björkman, J.W. (1989) Politicians, medicine and medicalising politics: physician power in the United States, in G. Freddi and J.W. Björkman (eds), *Controlling medical professionals: the comparative politics of health governance.* London: Sage.

Bloor, M. (2001) On the consulting room couch with citizen science; a consideration of the sociology of scientific knowledge perspective on practitioner–patient relationships. *Medical Sociology News.* British Sociological Association. September: 19–40.

Blumenthal, D. (2002) Doctors in a wired world: can professionalism survive connectivity? *The Millbank Quarterly*, 80(3): 525–46.

Borzel, T.A. (1998) Organising Babylon: on the different conceptions of policy networks. *Public Administration*, 76(2): 253–74.

Bristol Royal Infirmary Inquiry (2000) The inquiry into the management of care of children receiving complex heart surgery at the Bristol Royal Infirmary. *Interim report. Removal and retention of human material.* London: Stationery Office.

British Association of Medical Managers, British Medical Association, Institute of Health Services Management, Royal College of Nursing (1993) *Managing clinical services: a consensus statement of principles for effective clinical management.* London: Institute of Health Services Management.

British Medical Association (1994) *Complementary medicine: new approaches to good practice.* Oxford: Oxford University Press.

British Medical Association, Academy of Medical Royal Colleges, Joint Consultants Committee (1998) *Making self-regulation work at the local level.* London: BMA.

British Medical Association, Central Consultants and Specialists Committee (1998) *Guidance on clinical directorates.* London: BMA.

British Medical Journal (1994) General Medical Council says it will watch curriculum reforms. [Editorial] *British Medical Journal,* 308: 361.

British Medical Journal (1998a) The dark side of medicine. [Editorial] *British Medical Journal,* 316: 1733.

British Medical Journal (1998b) All changed, changed utterly. [Editorial] *British Medical Journal,* 317: 1917–18.

Burrage, M., Jarausch, K. and Siegrist, H. (1990) An actor based framework for the study of professions, in M. Burrage and R. Torstendahl (eds), *Professions in theory and history: rethinking the study of professions.* London: Sage.

Butler, J. (1992) *Patients, policies and politics.* Buckingham: Open University Press.

Calman, K. (1994) *Continuing medical education.* [Consultation Paper] London: Department of Health.

Campbell, S., Roland, M. and Wilkin, D. (2001) Improving the quality of care through clinical governance. *British Medical Journal,* 322: 1580–2.

Campbell, S., Sheaff, R., Sibbald, B., Marshall, M.N., Pickard, S., Gask, L., Halliwell, S., Rogers, A. and Roland, M.O. (2002) Implementing clinical governance in English primary care groups/trusts: reconciling quality improvement and quality assurance. *Quality and Safety in Health Care,* 11(1): 9–14.

Carlisle, D. (2003a) Patient choice 'gaming' leaves NHS beds empty. *Health Service Journal,* 24 July: 5.

Carlisle, D. (2003b) Change of heart. *Health Service Journal,* 15 May: 12–13.

Catto, G. (2001) Education, education, education. … *British Medical Journal,* 322: S2–7301.

Central Office for Research Ethics Committees (2001) *Governance arrangements for NHS Research Ethics Committees (GAfREC).* London: Department of Health.

Central Office for Research Ethics Committees (2002). http://www.corec.org.uk.

Chant, A.D.B. (1984) Practising doctors should not manage. *Lancet,* 1(8391): 1398.

Chantler, C. (1990) Managerial reform in a London hospital, in N. Carle (ed.), *Managing for health result.* London: King Edward's Hospital Fund for London, 74–85.

Chief Medical Officer (2001) *The removal, retention and use of human organs and tissue from post-mortem examinations.* London: Department of Health.

Chief Medical Officer's Review Group (1995) *Maintaining medical excellence: review of guidance on doctors' performance*. London: Department of Health.

Chisolm, J. (1999) Viagra: a botched test case for rationing. *British Medical Journal*, 318: 273–4.

Chrubasik, S., Junck, H., Sappe, H.A. and Stutzke, O. (1998) A survey on pain complaints and health care utilisation in a German population sample. *European Journal of Anaesthesiology*, 15: 397–408.

Clarke, J. and Newman, J. (1997) *The managerial state: power, politics and ideology in the remaking of social welfare*. London: Sage.

Coburn, S. (1993) State authority, medical dominance and trends in the regulation of the health professions: the Ontario case. *Social Science and Medicine*, 37(7): 841–50.

Coleman, W.D. (1999) Internationalised policy environments and policy network analysis. *Political Studies*, 47(4): 691–713.

Commission for Health Improvement (2001) *A guide to clinical governance reviews in NHS Trusts*. London: Commission for Health Improvement.

Committee on Publication Ethics (1999) *The COPE report 1999*. London: BMJ Publications.

Competition Commission (2000) *British United Provident Association Limited and Community Hospitals Group plc: a report on the proposed merger*. Cm 5003. London: Stationery Office.

Conference of Postgraduate Medical Deans of the UK (2002) *A guide to the management and quality assurance of postgraduate medical and dental education*. [Green Guide] London: Conference of Postgraduate Medical Deans of the UK.

Conrad, P. and Schneider, J. (1985) *Deviance and medicalisation: from badness to sickness*. London: Merrill.

Cooper, L.A. and Roter, D.L. (2002) Patient–provider communication: the effect of race and ethnicity on process and outcomes of health care, in Board on Health Sciences Policy, Division of Health Sciences Policy, Institute of Medicine, *Unequal treatment: confronting racial and ethnic disparities in health care* (pp. 552–93). Washington, DC: National Academies Press.

Coulter, A. (2002) *The autonomous patient. Ending paternalism in medical care*. London: Nuffield Trust.

Dauphinee, W.D. (1999) Revalidation of doctors in Canada. *British Medical Journal*, 319: 1188–90.

Davies, H.T., Hodges, C. and Rundal, T.G. (2003) Views of doctors and managers on the doctor–manager relationship. *British Medical Journal*, 326: 626–8.

Dawson, S.J.N. (1994) Changes in the distance. Professionals reappraise the meaning of management. *Journal of General Management*, 20: 1–21.

Day, P. and Klein, R. (1992) Constitutional and distributional conflict in British medical politics: the case of general practice, 1911–91. *Political Studies*, 40: 462–78.

Day, P. and Klein, R. (2001) *Auditing the auditors.* London: Stationery Office/Nuffield Trust.

Day, P. and Klein, R. (2002) Who nose best. *Health Service Journal,* 4 April: 27.

Department of Health (1989a) *Working for patients.* CM 555, London: HMSO.

Department of Health (1989b) *NHS consultants: appointments, contracts and distinction awards.* Working for Patients, Working Paper 7 London: HMSO.

Department of Health (1989c) *Implications for Family Practitioner Committees.* Working for Patients, Working Paper 8. London: HMSO.

Department of Health (1989d) *Indicative prescribing budgets for general medical practitioners.* Working for Patients, Working Paper 4. London: HMSO.

Department of Health (1989e) *Practice budgets for general medical practitioners.* Working for Patients, Working Paper 3. London: HMSO.

Department of Health (1990a) *Consultant contracts and job plans.* HC(90)16, London: Department of Health.

Department of Health (1990b) *Disciplinary procedures for hospital and community medical and dental staff.* HC(90)9, London: Department of Health.

Department of Health (1991) *Local research ethics committees.* HSG (91)5, London: Department of Health.

Department of Health (1992) *The Patient's Charter.* London: HMSO.

Department of Health (1994a) *Hospital medical and dental staff (England and Wales), terms and conditions of service.* London: Department of Health.

Department of Health (1994b) *Standards for local research ethics committees – a framework for ethical review.* London: Department of Health.

Department of Health (1995) *The Patient's Charter and You.* London: HMSO.

Department of Health (1997a) *The new NHS: modern, dependable.* White Paper. Cm 3807, London: Stationery Office.

Department of Health (1997b) *NHS priorities and planning guidance 1998/99.* EL(97)39, London: Department of Health.

Department of Health (1997c) *Ethics committee review of multi-centre research.* London: Department of Health.

Department of Health (1998a) NHS to have legal duty of ensuring quality for first time. *Press Release 98/141,* 13 April, London: Department of Health.

Department of Health (1998b) *A first class service: quality in the new NHS.* London: Department of Health.

Department of Health (1999a) *Supporting doctors, protecting patients.* A consultation paper on preventing, recognising and dealing with poor clinical performance of doctors in the NHS in England. London: Department of Health.

Department of Health (1999b) *Regulating private and voluntary health-care.* London: Department of Health.

Department of Health (2000a) *An organisation with a memory.* Report of an expert group on learning from adverse events in the NHS chaired by the CMO. London: Stationery Office.

Department of Health (2000b) *The NHS Plan.* London: Stationery Office.

Department of Health (2000c) *A health service of all the talents.* Consultation document on the review of workforce planning. London: Department of Health.

Department of Health (2000d) Central Office for Research Ethics Committees. Letter from Sir John Pattison to MREC and LREC chairmen and administrators, 31 August, London: Department of Health.

Department of Health (2000e) *Patient and public involvement in the new NHS.* London: Department of Health.

Department of Health (2001a) *Assuring the quality of medical practice. Implementing 'Supporting doctors, protecting patients'.* London: Department of Health.

Department of Health (2001b) *Research governance framework for health and social care.* London: Department of Health.

Department of Health (2001c) *Research governance implementation plan.* London: Department of Health.

Department of Health (2001d) *The NHS Plan. Proposal for a new approach to the consultant contract.* London: Department of Health.

Department of Health (2001e) *Rewarding commitment and excellence in the NHS. Proposals for a new consultant award scheme.* Consultation document. London: Department of Health.

Department of Health (2001f) *2001/2002: Arrangements for whole system capacity planning.* HSC 2001/014, London: Department of Health.

Department of Health (2001g) *Postgraduate medical education and training. The Medical Education Standards Board.* A paper for consultation. London: Department of Health.

Department of Health (2001h) *A Health Service of all the talents: results of consultation.* London: Department of Health.

Department of Health (2001i) *Building a safer NHS for patients. Implementing an organisation with a memory.* London: Department of Health.

Department of Health (2001j) *The Government's expenditure plans 2001–02 to 2003–04.* Cm 5103, London: Stationery Office.

Department of Health (2002a) Independent Safety Organisation welcomes government response to Kennedy Report. *Press Release.* 18 January, London: Department of Health.

Department of Health (2002b) *Delivering the NHS plan.* Cm 5503 London: Stationery Office.

Department of Health (2002c) *The NHS Plan: next steps for investment, next steps for reform.* London: Department of Health.

Department of Health (2002d) *Reform of the General Medical Council.* A paper for consultation. London: Department of Health.

Department of Health (2002e) NHS Foundation Hospitals to be freed from Whitehall control. Speech by Alan Milburn. *Press Release* 2002/0240, 22 May, London: Department of Health.

Department of Health (2002f) *Growing capacity. A new role for external healthcare providers in England.* London: Department of Health.

Department of Health (2002g) *The Government's response to the House of Commons Health Committee's First Report on the role of the private sector in the NHS.* Cm 5567, London: Stationery Office.

Department of Health (2002h) *Unfinished business: proposals for reform of the Senior House Officer grade.* A paper for consultation. London: Department of Health.

Department of Health (2002i) *Shifting the balance of power: the next steps.* London: Department of Health.

Department of Health (2002j) *Human bodies, human choices. The law on human organs and tissues in England and Wales.* Consultation report. London: Department of Health.

Department of Health (2002k) *Postgraduate medical education and training.* The Postgraduate Medical Education and Training Board. Statement on policy. London: Department of Health.

Department of Health (2003a) New streamlined training for junior doctors. *Press Release.* 2003/0078. 25 February, London: Department of Health.

Department of Health (2003b) *The Isaacs Report.* London: Department of Health.

Department of Health (2003c) *Terms and conditions – consultants (England).* London: Department of Health.

Departments of Health and General Medical Council (2002) URL: http://www.revalidation.uk.info

Department of Health and the Independent Healthcare Association (2000) *For the benefit of patients. A Concordat with the private and voluntary health care provider sector.* London: Department of Health.

Department of Health and Social Security (1972) *Management arrangements for the reorganised Health Service.* London: HMSO.

Department of Health and Social Security (1975) *Supervision of the ethics of clinical research investigations and foetal research.* HSC(IS)153, London: Department of Health and Social Security.

Department of Health and Social Security (1982) *Prevention of harm to patients resulting from physical or mental disability of hospital or community medical or dental staff.* HC(82)13, London: HMSO.

Department of Health and Social Security (1983a) *The NHS management inquiry.* Griffiths Report, London: HMSO.

Department of Health and Social Security (1983b) *Medical Act 1983.* London: HMSO.

Department of Health and Social Security (1986) *Health services management: Resource Management (Management Budgeting) in Health Authorities.* Circular HN(86)34, London: HMSO.

Department of Health and Social Security (1987) Steering group for implementation on behalf of the UK Health Departments, the Joint consultants Committee, and chairmen of Regional Health Authorities. *Achieving a balance: plan for action.* London: Department of Health and Social Security.

Dewar, S. and Finlayson, B. (2001) Reforming the GMC. *British Medical Journal,* 322: 689–90.

Dohler, M. (1989) Physicians' professional autonomy in the Welfare State: endangered or preserved? in G. Freddi and J.W. Bjorkman (eds), *Controlling medical professionals: the comparative politics of health governance* (pp. 178–97). London: Sage.

Donaldson, L. (1995) The listening blank. *Health Service Journal,* 21 September: 22–3.

Donaldson, L.J. (1994a) Doctors with problems in the NHS workforce. *British Medical Journal,* 308: 1277–82.

Donaldson, L.J. (1994b) Sick doctors: a responsibility to act. *British Medical Journal,* 309: 557–8.

Doyle, Y. and Bull, A. (2000) Role of private sector in United Kingdom healthcare system. *British Medical Journal,* 321: 563–5.

du Boulay, C. (2000) From CME to CPD: getting better at getting better? *British Medical Journal,* 320: 393–4.

Dunleavy, P. (1981) Professions and policy change: notes towards a model of ideological corporatism. *Public Administration Bulletin,* 36: 3–16.

Dunleavy, P. and O'Leary, B. (1987) *Theories of the state: the politics of liberal democracy.* London: Macmillan.

Edelman, M. (1985) Political language and political reality. *Political Studies,* 18(1), 10–19.

Edelman, M. (1988) *Constructing the political spectacle.* Chicago University Press: Chicago, IL.

Edwards, N. and Marshall, M. (2003) Doctors and managers. *British Medical Journal,* 326: 116–7.

Eisenberg, D.M., Davis, R.B., Ettner, S.L., Appel, S. *et al.* (1998) Trends in alternative medicine use in the United States, 1990–97. *Journal of the American Medical Association,* 280(18): 1569–75.

Elston, M.A. (1991) The politics of professional power: medicine in a changing health service, in J. Gabe, M. Calnan and M. Bury (eds), *The sociology of the Health Service.* London: Routledge.

Elwell, H. (1986) *NHS, the road to recovery.* London: Centre for Policy Studies.

Erichsen, V. (1995a) Health care reform in Norway: the end of the 'profession' state? *Journal of Health Politics, Policy and Law,* 20(3): 719–37.

Erichsen, V. (1995b) State traditions and medical professionals in Scandinavia, in T. Johnson, G. Larkins and M. Saks (eds), *Health professions and the state in Europe.* London: Routledge.

Ernst, E., Resch, K.L. and Hill, S. (1997) Do complementary practitioners have a better bedside manner than physicians? *Journal of the Royal Society of Medicine,* 90: 118–19.

Ernst, E. (1999) Complementary medicine: too good to be true? *Journal of the Royal Society of Medicine,* 92(1): 1–2.

Ernst, E. (2000) Herbal medicines: where is the evidence? *British Medical Journal*, 321: 395–6.

Evans, I. (1998) Conduct unbecoming – the MRC's approach. *British Medical Journal*, 316: 1728–9.

Exworthy, M. (1998) Clinical audit in the NHS internal market: from peer review to external monitoring. *Public Policy and Administration*, 13: 40–53.

Fairfield, G., Hunter, D.J., Mechanic, D. and Rosleff, F. (1997) Managed care; origins, principles and evolution. *British Medical Journal*, 314: 1823–6.

Falkum, E. and Førde, R. (2001) Paternalism, patient autonomy, and moral deliberation in the physician–patient relationship: attitudes with Norwegian physicians. *Social Science and Medicine*, 52: 239–48.

Ferrera, M. (1989) The politics of health reform: origins and performance of the Italian Health Service in comparative perspective, in G. Freddi and J.W. Bjorkman (eds), *Controlling medical professionals: the comparative politics of health governance* (pp. 116–29). London: Sage.

Ferlie, E., Ashburner, L. and Fitzgerald, L. (1996) *The new public management in action*. Oxford: Oxford University Press.

Ferriman, A. Report suggests that NHS is unsustainable in present form. *British Medical Journal*, 319: 801

Flynn, R. (1992) *Structures of control in health management*. London: Routledge.

Foster, A. (1991) *FHSAs: today's and tomorrow's priorities*. Leeds: National Health Service Management Authority.

Foster, C.G., Marshall, T. and Moodie P. (1995) The annual reports of local research ethics committees. *Journal of Medical Ethics*, 21: 214–19.

Foucault, M. (1973) *The birth of the clinic. An archaeology of medical perception*. London: Tavistock.

Foucault, M. (1977) *Discipline and punish: the birth of the prison*. London: Allen Lane.

Freddi, G. (1989) Problems of organisational rationality in health systems: political controls and policy options, in G. Freddi and J.W. Björkman (eds), *Controlling medical professionals: the comparative politics of health governance*. London: Sage.

Freidson, E. (1988) *The profession of medicine: a study of the sociology of applied knowledge*. London: University of Chicago Press.

Fulder, S. (1988) *The handbook of complementary medicine*. Oxford: Oxford University Press.

Furnham, A. and Smith, C. (1988) Choosing alternative medicine: a comparison of the beliefs of patients visiting a general practitioner and a homeopath. *Social Science and Medicine*, 26(7): 685–9.

Gamble, A. (1988) *The free economy and the strong state*. London: Macmillan.

General Medical Council, Education Committee (1987) *Recommendations on the training of specialists*. London: General Medical Council.

General Medical Council (1993) *Professional conduct and discipline: fitness to practice*. London: General Medical Council.

General Medical Council (1995) *Good medical practice.* London: General Medical Council.

General Medical Council (1997a) *When your performance is questioned.* London: General Medical Council.

General Medical Council (1997b) *The management of doctors with problems: referral to the GMC's fitness to practise procedures.* London: General Medical Council.

General Medical Council (1999a) *News.* Spring, Issue 5. London: General Medical Council.

General Medical Council (1999b) *Report of the revalidation steering group.* London: General Medical Council.

General Medical Council (2000) *Revalidating doctors. Ensuring standards, securing the future.* London: General Medical Council.

General Medical Council (2001) *Protecting patients: a summary consultative document.* London: General Medical Council.

General Medical Council (2002a) *Tomorrow's doctors, recommendations on undergraduate medical education.* London: General Medical Council.

General Medical Council (2002b) *Research: the roles and responsibilities of doctors.* London: General Medical Council.

Giaimo, S. (1995) Health care reform in Britain and Germany: recasting the political bargain with the medical profession. *Governance,* 8(3): 354–79.

Giddens, A. (1991) *Modernity and self-identity: self and society in the late modern age.* Cambridge: Polity Press.

Giddens, A. (1994) *Beyond left and right.* Cambridge: Polity Press.

Giddings, A. (1995) *Parliamentary accountability. A study of parliament and executive agencies.* Basingstoke: Macmillan.

Gill, V. (1998) Doing attributions in medical interaction: Patients' explanations for illness and doctors' responses. *Social Psychological Quarterly,* 61(6): 342–60.

Glennerster, H., Matsaganis, M. and Owens, P. (1994) *Implementing GP Fundholding.* Buckingham: Open University Press.

Goddard, M. and Sussex, J. (2002) Long-term aims and short-term realities; the impact of the NHS/private sector concordat. *Applied Health Economics and Health Policy,* 1(4): 165–9.

Goldstein, M. (1992) *The health movement; promoting fitness in America.* New York: Twayne.

Gray, J.A.M. (2002) *The resourceful patient.* Oxford: Rosetta Press.

Green, D. (1986) *Challenge to the NHS.* Hobart Paperback no. 23, London: Institute of Economic Affairs.

Green, D. (1988) *Everyone a private patient.* Hobart Paperback no. 27, London: Institute of Economic Affairs.

Greenwood, L. (2000) Barking mad. *Health Service Journal,* 13 July: 18.

Griffiths, L. and Hughes, D. (2000) Talking contracts and taking care: managers and professionals in the British National Health Service internal market. *Social Science and Medicine,* 51: 209–22.

Grossman, J.H. (1990) Physicians as managers in hospitals, in D. Costain (ed.), *The future of acute services: doctors as managers.* London: Kings Fund Centre for Health Services Development.

Gulland, A. (2001) Trust defends decision to retain private beds at Heart Hospital. *British Medical Journal,* 323: 358.

Gulland, A. (2003) Blair says whole of NHS should be opened up to competition. *British Medical Journal,* 326: 1106.

Gunn, L. (1978) Why is implementation so difficult? *Management services in government,* 33: 169–76.

Habermas, J. (1985) *The theory of communicative action.* Cambridge: Polity Press.

Hall, D. (1991) The research imperative and bureaucratic control: the case of clinical research. *Social Science and Medicine,* 32(3): 333–42.

Ham, C. (1985) *Health policy in Britain.* Basingstoke: Macmillan Education.

Harrison, S. and Dowswell, G. (2002) Autonomy and bureaucratic accountability in primary care: what general practitioners say. *Sociology of Health and Illness,* 24(2): 208–26.

Harrison, S. and Mort, M. (1998) Which champions, which people? Public and user involvement in health care as a technology of legitimation. *Social Policy and Administration,* 32(1): 60–70.

Harrison, S. and Pollitt, C. (1994) *Controlling health professionals: the future of work and organisation in the NHS.* Buckingham: Open University Press.

Harrison, S., Hunter, D.J., Marnoch, G. and Pollitt, C. (1992) *Just managing: power and culture in the National Health Service.* London: Macmillan.

Harrison, S., Hunter, D.J., Marnoch, G. and Pollitt, C.J. (1989) *The impact of general management in the NHS.* Leeds: Nuffield Institute.

Haug, M. (1973) Deprofessionalisation: an alternative hypothesis for the future. *Sociological Review Monograph,* 20: 195–211.

Haug, M. (1988) A re-examination of the hypothesis of professionalisation. *The Millbank Quarterly,* 66, supplement 2: 48–56.

Haug, M. and Levin, B. (1981) Practitioner or patient. Who's in charge? *Journal of Health and Social Behaviour,* 22: 212–29.

Haug, M. and Levin, B. (1983) *Consumerism in medicine; challenging physician authority.* London: Sage.

Havard, J. (1989) Advertising by doctors and the public interest. *British Medical Journal,* 298: 903.

Haywood, S. and Hunter, D. (1982) Consultative processes in health policy in the UK: a view from the centre. *Public Administration,* 69: 143–62.

Health Service Journal (2002) Here to stay. *Health Service Journal,* 30 May: 12.

Health Service Journal (2003) Battle 'lost' on private work. *Health Service Journal,* 30 January: 7.

Hindmoor, A. (1998) The importance of being trusted: transaction costs and policy network theory. *Public Administration,* 76(1): 25–44.

Hogg, C. (1999) *Patients, power and politics.* London: Sage.

Hood, C. (1991) A public management for all seasons? *Public Administration,* 69(1): 3–19.

Hopkins, P. (1972) *Patient-centred medicine.* London: Regional Doctor Publication.

Hopton, J.L. and Dlugolecka, M. (1995) Need and demand for primary health care: a comparative survey approach. *British Medical Journal,* 310: 1369–73.

Horton, R. (1998) UK medicine: what are we to do? *The Lancet,* 352: 1166.

House of Commons Select Committee on Health (1999) *The regulation of private and other independent healthcare.* Session 1998–99, Fifth Report, London: Stationery Office.

House of Commons Select Committee on Health (2000) *Consultant contracts* Session 1999–2000, Third Report, London: Stationery Office.

House of Commons Select Committee on Health (2002) *The role of the private sector in the NHS.* Session 2001–02, First Report, London: Stationery Office.

House of Commons Select Committee on Health (2003) *Patient and public involvement in the NHS.* Session 2002–03, Seventh Report, London: Stationery Office.

Hughes, G., Mears, R. and Winch, C. (1997) An inspector calls? Regulation and accountability in three public services. *Policy and Politics,* 25(3): 299–312.

Hunter, D.J. (1984) Consensus management or chief executives? Lessons from the NHS. *Local Government Studies,* 10: 39–50.

Hunter, D.J. (1991) Managing medicine: a response to the crisis. *Social Science and Medicine,* 32(4): 441–8.

Hunter, D. (1994) From tribalism to corporatism: the managerial challenge to medical dominance, in J. Gabe, D. Kelleher and G. Williams (eds), *Challenging medicine.* London: Routledge.

Iglehart, J.K. (1994) Physicians and the growth of managed care. Health policy report. *New England Journal of Medicine,* 331: 1167–71.

Institute of Health Services Management (1990) *Models of clinical management.* London: IHSM.

Institute of Healthcare Management (2002) NHS managers keep quiet rather than tell it how it is. *Press Release,* 9 October.

Irvine, Sir D. (1999) The performance of doctors: the new professionalism. *The Lancet,* 353: 1174–77.

Irvine, Sir D. (2000) Update on revalidation. *Journal of the Royal College of Physicians,* 34: 415–17.

Jasanoff, W. and Wynne, B. (1998) Science and decision making, in S. Rayner and E.L. Malone (eds), *Human choice and climate change. Vol 1: The societal framework* (pp. 1–87). Columbus, OH: Batelle Press.

Jones, J. (1999) UK watchdog issues guidelines to combat medical research fraud. *British Medical Journal,* 319: 660.

Jones, K., Baggott, R. and Allsop, J. (2000) Under the influence. *Health Service Journal,* 16 November, 28–9.

Keen, J. (2000) Private health care: modernisation stops here. *British Medical Journal*, 320: 202.

Kelleher, D. (1994) Self-help groups and their relationship to medicine, in J. Gabe, D. Kelleher and G. Williams (eds), *Challenging medicine* (pp. 104–17). London: Routledge.

Kelner, M. and Wellman, B. (1997) Health care and consumer choice: medical and alternative therapies. *Social Science and Medicine*, 45(2): 203–12.

Kent, G. (1997) The views of members of Local Research Ethics Committees, researchers and members of the public towards the roles and functions of LRECs. *Journal of Medical Ethics*, 23: 186–90.

Keogh, B.E. Dussek, J., Watson, D., Magee, P. and Wheatley, D. (1998) Public confidence and cardiac surgical outcome. *British Medical Journal*, 306: 1759–60.

Kerrison, S., Packwood, T. and Buxton, M. (1993) Monitoring medical audit, in R. Robinson and J. Le Grand (eds), *Evaluating the NHS reforms* (pp. 155–78). London: Kings Fund Institute.

Kingdon, J. (1984) *Agendas, alternatives and public policy*. Boston, MA: Little Brown.

Klein, R. (1989) *The politics of the NHS*. London: Longman.

Klein, R. (1990) The state and the profession: the politics of the double bed. *British Medical Journal*, 301: 700–2.

Klein, R. (1993) O'Goffe's tale', in C. Jones (ed.), *New perspectives on the welfare state in Europe* (pp. 7–17). London: Routledge.

Klein, R. (1995) Big bang health care reform – does it work? The case of Britain's 1991 National Health Service reforms. *Millbank Quarterly*, 73(3): 301–37.

Klein, R. (1998) Competence, self-regulation and the public interest. *British Medical Journal*, 301: 1740–42.

Kmietowicz, Z. (2003) Consultants vote in favour of revised contract. *British Medical Journal*, 327: 945.

Laing and Buisson (1995) *Laing's review of private healthcare 1995*. London: Laing and Buisson Publications.

Laing and Buisson (1996) *Laing's review of private healthcare 1996*. London: Laing and Buisson Publications.

Laing and Buisson (2002) *Laing's healthcare market review 2002–2003*. London: Laing and Buisson Publications.

Larkin, G. (1995) State control and the health professions in the United Kingdom, in T. Johnson, G. Larkin and M. Saks (eds), *Health professions and the state in Europe*. London: Routledge.

Laurent, C. (2000) With complements. *Health Service Journal*, 29 June: 18.

Lee-Potter, J. (1997) *A damned bad business: the NHS deformed*. London: Victor Gollancz.

Leese, B. and Bosanquet, N. (1995) Family doctors and change in practice strategy since 1986. *British Medical Journal*, 310: 705–8.

Letwin, O. and Redwood, J. (1988) *Britain's biggest enterprise: ideas for reform of the NHS*. London: Centre for Policy Studies.

Light, D. (2000) The two-tier system behind waiting lists. *British Medical Journal,* 320: 1349.

Limb, M. (2002) Erecting the barricades. Are English surgeons sabotaging government plans to use foreign teams to cut waiting lists? *British Medical Journal,* 325: 1262.

Lupton, D. (1994) *Medicine as culture: illness, disease and the body in Western societies.* London: Sage.

Lupton, D. (1997) Consumerism, reflexivity and the medical encounter. *Social Science and Medicine,* 45(3): 373–81.

MacDonald, S. (2003) Doctors are servants of patients, says CMO. *British Medical Journal,* 326: 1291–2.

MacLennan, A.H., Wilson, D.H. and Taylor, A.W. (1996) Prevalence and cost of alternative medicine in Australia. *Lancet,* 347: 569–73.

Marshall, T.H. (1950) *Citizenship and social class.* Cambridge: Cambridge University Press.

Marsh, D. and Smith, M. (2000) Understanding policy networks: towards a dialectical approach. *Political Studies,* 48(1): 4–21.

McCarthy, M. (1989) Introduction, in M. McCarthy (ed.), *The new politics of welfare.* Basingstoke: Macmillan.

McCombs, M.E. and Shaw, D.L. (1972) The agenda setting function of the mass media. *Public Opinion Quarterly,* 36: 176–87.

Mechanic, D. (1995) Dilemmas in rationing health care services: the case for implicit rationing. *British Medical Journal,* 310: 1655–9.

Medical Research Council (1997) *MRC policy and procedure for inquiring into allegations of scientific misconduct.* London: Medical Research Council.

Merrison Committee (1975). *Report of the inquiry into the regulation of the medical profession* (Chair, Sir Alec Merrison). Cmnd 6018. London: HMSO.

Milewa, T., Valentine, J. and Calnan, M. (1998) Managerialism and active citizenship in Britain's reformed health service: power and community in an era of decentralisation. *Social Science and Medicine,* 47(4): 507–17.

Millar, B. (1991) Clinicians as managers: medics make their minds up. *Health Service Journal,* 21 February: 17.

Millar, W.J. (1997) Use of alternative health care practitioners by Canadians. *Canadian Journal of Public Health,* 88: 154–8.

Monopolies and Mergers Commission (1993) *Private medical services: a report on agreements and practices relating to charges for the supply of private medical services by NHS consultants.* London: HMSO.

Mooney, H. (2003) Doctors shun leadership. *Health Service Journal,* 15 May: 10–11.

Moore, A. (2003) Partners in time. *Health Service Journal,* 24 April: 12–13.

Moran, M. (1999) *Governing the health care state. A comparative study of the United Kingdom, the United States, and Germany.* Manchester: Manchester University Press.

Moran, M. and Wood, B. (1993) *States, regulation and the medical profession*. Buckingham: Open University Press.

National Audit Office (1995) *Clinical audit in England*. HC 27, Session 1995–96. London: Stationery Office.

National Clinical Assessment Authority (2001a) *Business Plan 2001–02*. London: National Clinical Assessment Authority.

National Clinical Assessment Authority (2001b). *Information about the NCCA. Interim memorandum of understanding between the NCCA and the CHI*. URL: www.ncaa.nhs.uk/about/main.htm.

National Health Service Executive (1992) *Local voices: the views of local people in purchasing for health*. Leeds: National Health Service Executive.

National Health Service Executive (1994a) *Developing NHS purchasing and GP Fundholders*. EL(94)79. Leeds: National Health Service Executive.

National Health Service Executive (1994b) *Towards a primary care led NHS: an accountability framework for GP Fundholding*. EL(94)92. Leeds: National Health Service Executive.

National Health Service Executive (1996) *Clinical guidelines: using clinical guidelines to improve patient care within the NHS*. Leeds: National Health Service Executive.

National Health Service Executive (1997) *The management of doctors with problems: guidance on the role of the NHS in the GMC's performance procedures and the rehabilitation of doctors*. Leeds: National Health Service Executive.

National Health Service Executive (1999a) *Clinical governance: quality in the new NHS*. HSC 1999/065. Leeds: National Health Service Executive.

National Health Service Executive (1999b) *The NHS Performance Assessment Framework*. Leeds: National Health Service Executive.

National Health Service Executive (1999c) *Faster access to modern treatment. How NICE appraisal will work*. Leeds: National Health Service Executive.

National Health Service Executive (1999e) *Involvement works. The second report of the Standing Group on Consumers in NHS Research*. Leeds: National Health Service Executive.

National Health Service Executive, West Midlands (2000) *Report of a review of the research framework in North Staffordshire Hospital NHS Trust*. URL: www.doh.gov.uk/wmro/northstaffs.htm (Chair: Professor Rod Griffiths).

National Health Service Management Executive (1991a) *Priorities and planning guidance for the NHS for 1992/93*. EL(91)103. Leeds: National Health Service Management Executive.

National Health Service Management Executive (1991b) *Integrating primary and secondary health care*. London: National Health Service Management Executive.

National Primary Care Research and Development Centre (2002) *Clinical governance: the impact of NSFs on quality of care for mental health problems and coronary heart disease*. Project report. URL: http:// www.npcrdc.man.ac.uk. Manchester: National Primary Care Research and Development Centre.

Newble, D., Paget, N. and Mclaren, B. (1999) Revalidation in Australia and new Zealand: the approach of the Royal Australian College of Physicians. *British Medical Journal*, 319: 1185–8.

Nicholson, R.H. (ed.) (1986) *Medical research with children: ethics, law and practice*. Oxford: Oxford University Press.

Nigenda, G. (1997) Doctors and corporatist politics: the case of the Mexican medical profession. *Journal of Health, Politics, Policy and Law*, 22(1): 73–99.

Norcini, J. (1994) Recertification in the medical specialties. *Academic Medicine*, 69: 90–4S.

Norcini, J. (1999) Recertification in the United States. *British Medical Journal*, 319: 1183–85.

Norcini, J. and Dawson-Saunders, E. (1994) Issues in re-certification in North America, in D. Newble, B. Jolly and R. Wakeford (eds), *The certification and re-certification of doctors: issues in the assessment of clinical competence*. Cambridge: Cambridge University Press.

Norcini, J. and Shea, J.A. (1997) Increasing pressures for re-certification and re-licensure, in L. Curry and J. Wergin (eds), *Educating professionals: responding to new expectations for competence and accountability*. San Francisco: Jossey-Bass.

Packwood, T., Buxton, M. and Keen, J. (1990) Resource Management in the National Health Service: a first case study. *Policy and Politics*, 18(4): 245–55.

Paice, E. and Goldberg, I. (1998) What do postgraduate deans do? *British Medical Journal*, 316: 2.

Pappworth, M.H. (1969) *Human guinea pigs*. London: Penguin Harmondsworth.

Parsons, R. (1951) *The social system*. Glencoe, IL: Free Press.

Pauluch, D., Cain, R. and Gillett, J. (1994) Ideology and alternative therapy use among people living with HIV/AIDs. *Health and Canadian Society*, 2(1): 63–84.

Pay and Workforce Research (1999) *Managing consultant private practice*. London: Pay and Workforce Research.

Pickworth, E. (2000) Should local research ethics committees monitor research they have approved? *Journal of Medical Ethics*, 26: 330–3.

Pollitt, C. (1990) *Managerialism and the public services*. Oxford: Blackwell.

Pollitt, C. (1993) The politics of medical quality: auditing doctors in the UK and the USA. *Health Services Management Research*, 6: 24–34.

Pope, C. (1992) Cutting queues or cutting corners: waiting lists and the 1990 NHS reforms. *British Medical Journal*, 305: 577–9.

Powell, J.A. (2002) The doctor, the patient and the world-wide web: how the internet is changing healthcare. *Journal of the Royal Society of Medicine*, 96: 74–6.

Protess, D.L. and McCombs, M. (eds) (1991) *Agenda setting: readings on media public opinion and policy making*. New Jersey: Lawrence Erlbaum Associates.

Ranson, S. and Stewart, J. (1989) Citizenship and government: the challenge for management in the public domain. *Political Studies*, 37: 5–24.

Rasmussen, N.K. and Morgall, J.M. (1990) The use of alternative treatments in the Danish adult population. *Complementary Medicine Research*, 4: 16–22.

Rennie, D. (1998) An American perspective on research integrity. *British Medical Journal*, 316: 1726–33.

Review Body on Doctors' and Dentists' Remuneration (2003) *Review for 2003. Written evidence from the Health Departments of Great Britain.* London: Department of Health.

Riley, W. (2003) Consultant appraisal is trying to achieve too much. *British Medical Journal*, 326: S162.

Roberts, C.A. and Aruguete, M.S. (2000) Task and socio-emotional behaviors of physicians: a test of reciprocity and social interaction theories in analogue physician–patient encounters. *Social Science and Medicine*, 50: 309–15.

Roberts, F. (2000) The interactional construction of asymmetry: the medical agenda as a resource for delaying response to patient questions. *The Sociological Quarterly*, 41(1): 151–71.

Robinson, J. (1999) The price of deceit: the reflections of an advocate in M.M. Rosenthal, L. Mulcahy and S. Lloyd-Bostock, *Medical mishaps: pieces of the puzzle* (pp. 250–1). Buckingham: Open University Press.

Rodin, J. and Janis, I.L. (1979) The social power of health care practitioners as agents of social change. *Journal of Social Issues*, 35: 60–81.

Ross, E.C. (1999) Regulating managed care: interest group competition for control and behavioral health care. *Journal of Health, Politics and Law*, 24(3): 598–625.

Royal College of Anaesthetists and the Association of Anaesthetists of Great Britain and Ireland (1998) *Good practice: a guide for departments of anaesthia.* London: Royal College of Anaesthetists.

Royal College of General Practitioners (1999). *Revalidation and the RCGP.* London: Royal College of General Practitioners.

Royal College of Obstetricians and Gynaecologists (1998) *The Royal College of Obstetricians and Gynaecologists and clinical governance.* London: Royal College of Obstetricians and Gynaecologists.

Royal College of Obstetricians and Gynaecologists (2000a). Revalidation. URL: http://www.rcog.org.uk/ mainpages.asp? Page ID=437.

Royal College of Obstetricians and Gynaecologists (2000b) *Ethical guidelines.* London: Royal College of Obstetricians and Gynaecologists.

Royal College of Pathologists (2000) *Guidelines for the retention of tissues and organs at post-mortem examination.* London: Royal College of Pathologists.

Royal College of Physicians of London (1989) *Medical audit: a first report. What, why and how?* London: Royal College of Physicians of London.

Royal College of Physicians of London (1996) *Guidelines on the practice of ethics committees in medical research involving human subjects.* London: Royal College of Physicians of London.

Royal College of Physicians of London (1999) *Physicians maintaining good medical practice: clinical governance and self-regulation*. London: Royal College of Physicians of London.

Royal College of Psychiatrists (2000) *Guidelines for researchers and for research ethics committees on psychiatric research involving human participants*. London: Royal College of Psychiatrists.

Royal College of Surgeons of England (1988) Commission on the provision of surgical services. *Report of the working party on the composition of a surgical team – general surgery, orthopaedics and Otolaryngology*. London: Royal College of Surgeons of England.

Royal College of Surgeons of England (1989) *Guidelines to clinical audit in surgical practice*. London: Royal College of Surgeons of England.

Royal Liverpool Children's Hospital Inquiry (2001) *Summary and recommendations*. London: House of Commons.

Sabatier, P.A. (1988) An advocacy coalition framework of policy change and the role of policy-oriented learning therein. *Policy Sciences*, 21: 129–68.

Saks, M. (1995) *Professions and the public interest*. London: Routledge.

Salter, B. (1994) Change in the NHS: policy paradox and the rationing issue. *International Journal of Health Services*, 24(1): 45–72.

Salter, B. (1995) Medicine and the state: redefining the concordat. *Public Policy and Administration*, 10(3): 60–87.

Salter, B. (1998) *The politics of change in the Health Service*. Basingstoke: Macmillan.

Salter, B. (1999) Change in the governance of medicine: the politics of self-regulation. *Policy and Politics*, 27(2): 143–58.

Salter, B. (2000) *Medical regulation and public trust: an international review*. London: Kings Fund.

Salter, B. (2001) Who rules: the new politics of medical regulation. *Social Science and Medicine*, 52: 871–83.

Sang, B. (2000) The customer is sometimes right. *Health Service Journal*, 18 August: 22–3.

Saunders, P. (1993) Citizenship in a liberal society, in B.S. Turner (ed.), *Citizenship and social theory*. London: Sage Publications.

Saward, M. (1990) Co-option and power: who gets what from formal incorporation. *Political Studies*, 38: 588–602.

Schepers, R. (1995) The Belgium medical profession since the 1980s, dominance and decline? in T. Johnson, G. Larkin and M. Saks (eds), *Health professions and the state in Europe*. London: Routledge.

Schepers, R. and Casparie, A.F. (1997) Continuity or discontinuity in the self-regulation of the Belgium and Dutch medical professions. *Sociology of Health and Illness*, 19(5): 580–600.

Secretary of State for Health (2001) Royal Liverpool Children's Inquiry published today. Statement to the House of Commons. *Press Release 2001/0059*. 30 January.

Senate of Surgery of Great Britain and Ireland (1998) *Response to the General Medical Council determination on the Bristol case*. London: Senate of Surgery of Great Britain and Ireland.

Shackley, P. and Ryan, M. (1994) What is the role of the consumer in health care? *Journal of Social Policy*, 23(4): 517–41.

Shamash, J. (2002) Second coming. *Health Service Journal*, 4 April: 12.

Sharma, U. (1995) *Complementary medicine today: practitioners and patients*. London: Routledge.

Shipman Inquiry (2002a) *Death disguised*. First Report. London: Shipman Inquiry (Chair: Dame Janet Smith DBE).

Shipman Inquiry (2002b) *Developing a new system for death certification*. A discussion paper. London: Shipman Inquiry (Chair: Dame Janet Smith DBE).

Smith, M.J. (1991) From policy community to issue network: salmonella in eggs and the new politics of food. *Public Administration*, 69: 235–55.

Smith, R. (1995) The future of the GMC: an interview with Donald Irvine, the new president. *British Medical Journal*, 310: 1515–18.

Smith, R. (1998) The need for a national body for research misconduct. *British Medical Journal*, 316: 1687.

Smith, R. (2001) GMC: approaching the abyss. *British Medical Journal*, 322: 1196.

Smith, R. (2002) Take back your mink, take back your pearls. *British Medical Journal*, 325: 1047–8.

Smith, R. (2003) The failures of two contracts. *British Medical Journal*, 326: 1097–8.

Smith, T., Moore, E. and Tunstall-Pedoe, H. (1997) Review by a local medical research ethics committee of the conduct of approved research projects, by examination of patients' case notes, consent forms, and research records and by interview. *British Medical Journal*, 314: 1588.

Southgate, L. (1994) Freedom and discipline: clinical practice and the assessment of clinical competence. *British Journal of General Practice*, 44: 87–9.

Southgate, L. and Jolly, B. (1994) Determining the content of re-certification procedures, in D. Newble, B. Jolly and R. Wakeford (eds), *The certification and re-certification of doctors: issues in the assessment of clinical competence*. Cambridge: Cambridge University Press.

Spry, C. (1990) Clinical directorates: a management point of view, in D. Dostain (ed.), *The future of acute services: doctors as managers*. London: Kings Fund Centre for Health Service Development.

Stacey, M. (1984) The General Medical Council and professional accountability. *Public Policy and Administration*, 4(1): 12–27.

Stacey, M. (1985) Medical ethics and medical practice: a social science view. Paper presented to *International symposium on ethical issues in social research*. London.

Stacey, M. (1992a) *Regulating British medicine: the General Medical Council*. London: John Wiley.

Stacey, M. (1992b) For public or profession: the new GMC performance procedures. *British Medical Journal*, 305: 1085–7.

Stacey, M. (2000) The General Medical Council and Professional Self-regulation, in D. Gladstone (ed.), *Regulating doctors*. London: Institute for the Study of Civil Society, 28–39.

Starr, P. (1982) *The social transformation of American medicine.* New York: Basic Books.

Stephenson, P. (2003) London patient choice 'pays more than private'. *Health Service Journal,* 9 January: 6.

Stevens, R. (1966) *Medical practice in modern England. The impact of specialisation and state medicine.* New Haven: Yale University Press.

Stewart, J. (1998) Advance or retreat: from the traditions of public administration to the new public management and beyond. *Public Policy and Administration,* 13(4): 12–27.

Stewart, J. and Stoker, G. (1995) *Local government in the 1990s.* London: Macmillan.

Stewart, M., Brown, J.B., Weston, W., McWhinney, I.R., McWilliam., C.L. and Freeman, T.R. (1995) *Patient centred medicine: transforming the clinical method.* London: Sage.

Sullivan, R. (2000) Direct-to-consumer advertising: the future in Europe. *Journal of the Royal Society of Medicine,* 93: 400–1.

Sutherland, K. and Dawson, S. (1998) Power and improvement in the new NHS: the roles of doctors and managers. *Quality in Health Care,* 7(Supplement): S16–S23.

Sweet, M. (2003) Brandy, bridge and other patient dilemmas. *British Medical Journal,* 326: 1291–2.

Swinkels, J.A. (1999) Registration of medical specialists in the Netherlands. *British Medical Journal,* 319: 1191–2.

Titmuss, R. (1968) *Commitment to welfare.* London: Allen and Unwin.

Tomlin, Z. (1990) No manager is an island – nor is any doctor. *Health Service Journal,* 20 December: 13.

Transition Advisory Board (2002) *Patient and public involvement in health.* Interim report of the Transition Advisory Board to the Department of Health. London: Transition Advisory Board.

Trostle, J.A. (1988) Medical compliance as an ideology. *Social Science and Medicine,* 27(12): 1299–308.

Turner, S. (1995) NHSE study shows doctors are hostile to management. *British Medical Association News Review,* December: 13.

Vaskilampi, T., Meriläinen, P., Sinkkonen, S. *et al.* (1993) The use of alternative treatments in the Finnish adult population, in G.T. Lewith and D. Aldridge (eds), *Clinical research methodology for complementary therapies.* London: Hodder and Stoughton, 204–29.

Vincent, C. and Furnham, A. (1996) Why do patients turn to complementary medicine? An empirical study. *British Journal of Clinical Psychology,* 35: 37–48.

Walsh, K. (1995) *Public service and market mechanisms. Competition, contracting and the New Public Management.* Basingstoke: Macmillan.

Ward, S. (1994) Education for life. *News Review. British Medical Association,* September: 18–19.

Waters, J. (1995) Highland clearances. *Health Service Journal,* 16 November: 13.

Watkin, B. (ed.) (1975) *Documents on health and social services: 1834 to the present day.* London: Methuen.

West, R. (1993) Joining the queue: demand and decision making, in S. Frankel and R. West (eds), *Rationing and rationality in the NHS. The persistence of waiting lists.* Basingstoke: Macmillan, 47–66.

Wiles, R. and Higgins, J. (1992) *Why do patients go private? A study of consumerism in health care.* Southampton: Institute for Health Policy Studies.

Williams, S. and Calnan, M. (1996) The 'limits' of medicalization? Modern medicine and the lay populace in late modernity. *Social Science and Medicine*, 42(12): 1609–20.

Williams, G. and Popay, J. (1994) Lay knowledge and the privilege of experience, in J. Gabe, D. Kelleher and G. Williams (eds), *Challenging medicine* (pp. 118–39). London: Routledge.

Wilsford, D. (1991) *Doctors and the state: the politics of health care in France and the United States.* Durham and London: Duke University Press.

Wilson, S.M. (1999) Impact of the Internet on primary care staff in Glasgow. *Journal of Medical Internet Research*, 1: e7.

Wohl, S. (1984) *The medical industrial complex.* New York: Harmony Books.

Wood, B. (2000) *Patient power: the politics of patients' associations in Britain and America.* Buckingham: Open University Press.

Working Group on Specialist Medical Training (1993) *Hospital doctors: training for the future.* London: Department of Health [Calman Report].

Wright, M. (1988) Policy community, policy network and comparative industry policies, *Political Studies*, 36: 593–612.

Young, A. (1986) *Evaluating Management Budgeting in the NHS.* Glasgow: Young Consultants.

Zola, I.K. (1972) Medicine as an institution of social control. *Sociological Review*, 20(4): 487–504.

Zollman, C. and Vickers, A. (1999a) Users and practitioners of complementary medicine, *British Medical Journal*, 319: 836–8.

Zollman, C. and Vickers, A. (1999b) Complementary medicine and the patient, *British Medical Journal*, 319: 1486–9.

Zollman, C. and Vickers, A. (1999c) Complementary medicine in conventional practice, *British Medical Journal*, 319: 901–4.

Zollman, C. and Vickers, A. (1999d) Complementary medicine and the doctor, *British Medical Journal*, 319: 1558–61.

Index